Eighteenth-Century Dermatological Handbook

Eighteenth-Century Dermatological Handbook

Plenck's *Doctrina de Morbis Cutaneis*

Scott M. Jackson and Althea C. Ashe

ANTHEM PRESS

Anthem Press
An imprint of Wimbledon Publishing Company
www.anthempress.com

This edition first published in UK and USA 2026
by ANTHEM PRESS
75–76 Blackfriars Road, London SE1 8HA, UK
or PO Box 9779, London SW19 7ZG, UK
and
244 Madison Ave #116, New York, NY 10016, USA

British Library Cataloguing-in-Publication Data
A catalogue record for this book is available from the British Library.

Library of Congress Control Number: 2025926889

ISBN-13: 978-1-83999-936-9
ISBN-10: 1-83999-936-5

Cover credit: Photo of Scott Jackson's own copy of the 1783 edition of Doctrina de morbis cutaneis

This title is also available as an eBook.

CONTENTS

INTRODUCTION

"In science, the credit goes to the man who convinces the world, not to the man to whom the idea first occurs." – Sir Francis Darwin (1914) or Sir William Osler (1918)

Dermatology's origins as a specialty of medicine can be traced back to 1790 in London, 1801 in Paris, 1841 in Vienna, and 1869 in the United States. The founders of dermatology were individuals who decided the skin was worthy of their whole attention, and institutions were dedicated to this specialized study starting in the nineteenth century. For the most part, we should think of the nineteenth century as the century dermatology arrived. However, in 1776 an Austro-Hungarian surgeon named Joseph Jacob Plenck (1738–1807) unknowingly laid the foundation for the coming specialty with a handbook for his students entitled *Doctrina de Morbis Cutaneis,* which translates from the Latin to "Instruction on Skin Diseases." The work represents a major milestone along the way toward our modern view of skin disease. It contains the first scientific classification of skin diseases according to their appearance. The skin-focused physicians in the generation that followed the publication of this text—especially Robert Willan (1757–1812), widely considered the founder of the specialty of dermatology—built upon the knowledge contained within this foundational text.

Doctrina was not the first important work in the history of dermatology. It was preceded by three landmark publications: *De Morbis Cutaneis* (1572) by Hieronymus Mercurialis (1530–1606), *Pandocheion Aiolodermon* (1630) by Samuel Hafenreffer (1587–1660), and *De Morbis Cutaneis* (1714) by Daniel Turner (1667–1741). The Mercurialis text was the first work devoted to skin disease. Written in Latin, the lengthy Hafenreffer text—the Greek title of which translates roughly to "Compendium of Skin Affections"—was the second. The Turner text, with its deceiving Latin title, was the first work devoted to skin disease in English. In addition, the French physician Anne-Charles Lorry (1726–1783) released a verbose Latin treatise on skin disease (*Tractatus de Morbis Cutaneis*) a year after Plenck's *Doctrina* was released.

Beyond these significant works, there were innumerable texts that contained chapters focused on skin disease dating back to ancient times. The most critical of these texts include the fifth and sixth books of Celsus' multi-volume *De Medicina* (first century CE), Galen's *On Abnormal Swellings* (second century CE), the fourth book of Paul of Aegina's *Medical Compendium in Seven Books* (seventh century CE), and the fourth book of Avicenna's *Canon of Medicine* (1025). Other significant figures writing about the skin before the eighteenth century were Scribonius Largus (1–50 CE), Pliny the Elder (23–79 CE), Cassius Felix (fifth century CE), Alexander of Tralles (525–605 CE), Isidore of Seville (536–630 CE), Rhazes (865–935), Haly Abbas (tenth century), Hildegard of Bingen (1098–1179), Henri de Mondeville (1260–1320), Guy de Chauliac (1300–1368), Jan Jessen (1566–1621), Daniel Sennert (1572–1637), Jean Riolan the Younger (1577–1657), and Richard Wiseman (1622–1676).

Before the publication of *Doctrina*, knowledge related to the skin and its diseases had stagnated. Over the centuries, the contributors to the knowledge about the skin had produced page after page of information about the skin and its diseases, but the knowledge contained within those pages had not changed appreciably since ancient times. What now follows is a brief chronological summary of that knowledge, focusing on the Western medical tradition, which typically starts with the ancient Greeks and Romans.

The ancient Greeks viewed the skin as a fishnet-like envelope encasing the body, strong enough to protect the underlying structures and keep them contained, but porous enough to allow humors and other substances to seep out of the body. Humors are the four liquid substances (blood, phlegm, yellow bile, and black bile) that the body contains, and it was imbalances or corruption of one or more of these humors that they believed led to disease. Skin diseases such as psoriasis or eczema were widely considered to reflect quantitative or qualitative problems with these humors inside the body.

According to the ancient Greeks, the skin could not have its own diseases. The idea that the skin itself could be diseased was not suggested until 1601, and the anatomical basis for disease did not arrive until the eighteenth century. The Hippocratic corpus—that body of Greek medical texts from many different authors that was compiled in the fourth and third centuries BCE—did contain references to many different skin "affections," but the descriptions are lacking in detail and did not appear to be a main focus of these writers.

The Roman encyclopedist Aulus Cornelius Celsus (25 BCE–50 CE) brought much diagnostic clarity to the different skin diseases that the ancient physician faced in the first century CE. His descriptions of each disease were much more detailed and complete for the time. But his text was lost, and the benefit of any information contained within its pages was delayed for almost

1400 years. The most crucial of the ancient Roman physicians, Galen (129–216 CE), added knowledge about the skin's sensory function but failed to offer any new insights into skin disease. The first discussion of the psychological suffering caused by a skin disease (mentagra) was found in the *Historia Naturalis* of Pliny the Elder (23–79 CE). The Roman *medicus* certainly had more terms to choose to designate his patient's skin condition than did the Greeks. But by the end of the Roman era, there was much diagnostic confusion—some terms still in Greek, others in Latin, one term referring to different diseases, and multiple terms referring to the same disease. The meaning of dermatological terms from text to text was consistently inconsistent. Throughout this period, skin diseases remained a symptom of internal humoral imbalance, and they were treated with various methods which were believed to correct the imbalance, such as bloodletting and purging with various laxative substances.

The Middle Ages brought little change in the way skin diseases were viewed or treated, but there were a few bright spots—intellectually-speaking—in this fairly dark era that moved things forward slightly. The author of *Etymologies*, Isidore of Seville, attempted to clear up some of the terminological confusion by providing a seventh-century clear definition of terms in Latin. Several Byzantine physicians, including the aforementioned Paul of Aegina (625–690), compiled much of the ancient medical information of the Greeks and Romans and preserved it in several important Greek texts of the sixth and seventh centuries. While the Greek language was the primary language of medicine until the end of the Roman Empire, it was replaced with Latin in the early Middle Ages. Still, the information contained within these Byzantine Greek texts was important, and the ninth-century Arabic medical men realized this.

Starting in the ninth century, the Greek-to-Arabic translation movement developed in Baghdad. These works would later be translated into Latin in the twelfth and thirteenth centuries, thus securing the knowledge for all posterity via this translational progression from Greek to Arabic to Latin. The most impressive original work on skin disease appeared in the spectacular period of intellectual achievement—the best since Celsus' *De Medicina*—known as the Islamic Golden Age. That work was *Treatise on smallpox and measles* (circa 900) by Rhazes (865–925), in which the master medieval physician discussed in explicit detail the differences between the two eruptions, which were inexplicably confused at the time. The other celebrated medieval Arabic physician was Avicenna (980–1037), whose comprehensive overview of eleventh-century knowledge about skin disease was possibly the most referenced work on the subject in the history of medicine, having a long reign of 700 years as a primary medical textbook consulted by medical students of Europe as well as the Middle East.

In the medieval West, the responsibility of dealing with complaints of skin lesions was delegated to the surgeon, and surgical writers such as Henri de Mondeville (1260–1320) and Guy de Chauliac (1300–1368) recorded their own understanding of skin diseases, lamenting the diagnostic confusion that persisted at this time. The major scientific advancements in the medieval West regarding skin disease involved the increasing clarity regarding the diagnosis of leprosy, as the governments of Europe were forced to deal with the crisis brought about by a rise in prevalence of that disease (1 in 30 by the high Middle Ages). Still, many different skin diseases, notably psoriasis, were undoubtedly lumped under the diagnosis of lepra, and this confusion was not settled until the nineteenth century. The skin was viewed during the Middle Ages as an envelope with excretory and sensory functions, and its diseases remained "affections" resulting from humoral imbalance, corrected with the same balancing measures of the ancients: bloodletting and purging.

The Renaissance did not usher in a new way of thinking about the skin or its diseases. If anything, the "back to the sources" approach of the Renaissance humanist physician searching for medical information caused a rebirth of dated, Galenical methods of medicine. It was during this era that Mercurialis authored the aforementioned first text devoted to skin disease, but that text was merely an accumulation of all Galenical knowledge about skin disease, containing no new information. The only glimmer of modernity found in this period was presented by Jan Jessen (1566–1621), the first to suggest that the skin has its own diseases and that skin disease can be more than simply a reflection of internal humoral imbalances.

There were four important public health factors that drove an interest in skin disease in the sixteenth and seventeenth centuries: leprosy, plague, syphilis, and smallpox. Each of these diseases ravaged Europe during the Renaissance and had major skin manifestations; therefore, the skin was constantly on the mind of the European physician and surgeon. It was this fact that very likely spurred the medical community of this epoch to finally come to terms with the skin, a part of the body that had been largely ignored throughout history.

Laboratories became equipped with microscopes in the seventeenth century, with physician-scientists, such as Marcello Malpighi (1628–1694), able to see for the first time the skin's layers and structures. That invention, coupled with Bacon's scientific method and Harvey's discovery of blood circulation, began a wave of innovation in medicine that caused a significant degree of questioning of the ancients. The end result of the Scientific Revolution, known as the Enlightenment, was a complete rejection of the authority of the ancients and a new beginning in science, as well as in medicine. It was toward the end of this period that Plenck wrote *Doctrina de Morbis Cutaneis,* a book that would become the defining dermatological text of the Enlightenment.

Prior to the eighteenth century, skin diseases were organized ("classified" would be too strong a word to use at this point) with the same system used by the ancient Greek physician Galen: diseases of the scalp and diseases of the rest of the body. This simplified approach was very unimaginative and implies that the ancients did not think much about the diseases. There was a notion that diseases of hair-bearing areas were somehow different from those of the rest of the body. Hair was deemed to be composed of an excreted substance, and diseases of the hair were believed to be caused by some abnormality of this excretion from the body. Texts on skin disease, such as that by Mercurialis, followed suit with this system of organizing skin diseases.

There were two attempts at organizing skin diseases differently from Galen that ultimately did not capture the interest of medical writers at the time—or afterward. First was the system of the esteemed eleventh-century Arabic physician Avicenna, who discussed skin diseases in his famous fourth book of *Canon of Medicine* as "swellings," which he divided into hot swellings, cold swellings, and papular swellings. The other was the system of the seventeenth-century French physician Riolanus (1580–1657) who divided skin diseases into pustules, deformities, and tubercles. In spite of considerable referencing of both physicians by the medical writers who followed them, neither system demonstrated any staying power; diseases of the skin remained as chaotically arranged as they were in ancient times.

As mentioned previously, the scientific revolution first laid bare many of the flaws of the ancients, and the Enlightenment was the beginning of the end for the reign of the ancients in medicine. This latter period of intellectual achievement—roughly 1680s to 1790s—saw the first impulses to define and classify diseases (termed nosology) using observational and empirical data generated by practicing physicians with a penchant for new data and a tendency to reject old knowledge. A new nosology had been called for in the seventeenth century by Thomas Sydenham (1624–1689), who in many ways was the first physician of the modern era. Put forth by François Boissier de Sauvages de Lacroix (1706–1767), the first classification of disease appeared in 1731 in a title called *Nouvelles classes de maladies.* Shortly thereafter, the Swedish physician-naturalist Carl Linnaeus (1707–1778) produced his classification of living things in *Systema naturae* (1735), setting the standard for the way diseases would be classified during the Enlightenment. Sauvages and Linnaeus inspired numerous physician-botanists in the latter half of the eighteenth century to create their own systems of classification. The most significant of these was the Scottish Enlightenment dynamo William Cullen (1710–1790), along with other noteworthy nosologists of the era including Rudolf Augustin

Vogel (1724–1774), Johann Baptiste Michael Sagar (1702–1778), and David Macbride (1726–1778). According to the Plenck's preface to *Doctrina*, all of these writers inspired him to develop his own system for classifying skin diseases. Thus *Doctrina* was a direct consequence of the Enlightenment drive to classify everything. Now that we have introduced the text, let us take a closer look at its author.

The Author

Joseph Jacob Plenck was born in Vienna on November 28, 1735, the son of a bookbinder, Franz Plenck, and Maria Anna Pochtl. After attending the Jesuit Latin School, Plenck became an apprentice to Johann Christian Retter, a Viennese surgeon. In 1756 at 21 years of age, Plenck enrolled in the illustrious medical school at the University of Vienna, where he became a pupil of the generalist Anton de Häen (1704–1776) and the surgeon Ferdinand von Leber (1727–1808). Two years later, Plenck enlisted in the Imperial army, which was allied with England against Prussia and France in the Seven Years War. He served as regimental surgeon, only to return to his medical studies at the end of the war in 1764. Plenck sold his parental home in order to acquire office space and a license to practice surgery. He wed his first wife that year, Catherina Sophia Sartori, the daughter of a hospital administrator. His first child, Sebastian, was born a year later but died at four months of age; his second child and only daughter, Antonia, was born in 1767. Plenck's third child, a boy named Joseph, died after seventeen days. In 1770, Plenck was given his first professorship in Surgery and Obstetrics at the University of Basel.

Plenck's fame increased to the point that the Habsburg Empress, Maria Theresa, commissioned him in 1771 to join the faculty of a newly established university in Tyrnau, which was in Hungary at the time (now Trnava, Slovakia). His first wife died at some unknown point while Plenck was in Tyrnau. In 1777, the university was moved to Budapest, and Plenck transferred with it. Plenck remarried in 1779—to Franzisca Autrath—and had two sons: Gabriel (1779), who died soon after birth, and Johannes (1781). In 1783, he returned to Vienna to fill a vacant position of director of military pharmacies, and there he remained until his retirement. Three years later in 1786, Plenck was named professor of chemistry and botany at the Josephinum, the Medicochirurgical Military Academy established by Joseph II of Austria. The Josephinum was attached to the Allgemeines Krankenhaus, the Vienna General Hospital that had been established by Joseph a year earlier. In 1797, Plenck was knighted by Francis II as a knight of the kingdom of Hungary. In 1799, Plenck lost his only surviving son,

Johannes, at nineteen years of age. Plenck was granted retirement with full salary in 1805. He died two years later, having suffered the last years of his life with paraplegia. Plenck tragically outlived his four sons and two wives, survived only by his two daughters, Antonia and Anna, the latter born at an unknown time after 1781.

Plenck was perceived as a talented educator and a learned man. An anonymous writer who attended his lectures in 1793 wrote,

> Among the physicians in Vienna who deserve attention on account of their learning, Plenck and a few others at the Military Academy stand out. Plenck is distinguished by his industry and range of knowledge, a range which is unusual in a man of his age, in the field of the contemporary progress of knowledge. The hours I spent listening to him I count among the most pleasant and profitable spent in Vienna.[1]

Plenck's industry was unsurpassed by his fellow eighteenth-century physician writers. His first book appeared in 1767; the English translation of the title of this Latin work was *A New and Easy Method of Giving Mercury to Those Afflicted with the Venereal Disease: To Which is Annexed a New Theory of the Action of This Metal on the Salivary Glands.* That work contains a description of a gummy form of mercury which Plenck had invented, promising less salivation as a side effect compared to the more traditional forms of mercury. The salivation was a side effect one could not hide; rather than reveal this tell-tale sign of syphilis to the world, a person receiving mercurial treatment opted instead for hiding away at home for a month or longer while the treatment ensued. Plenck's new treatment was made by combining one part water, two parts gum acacia, and one part mercury. This mixture was eventually given the name *mercurius gummosus plenkii.* Plenck's gum was met with enthusiasm by his peers, but the consensus was that salivation did not fully cease with this version of mercury, although it was indeed less intense for some subjects. Regardless of whether the gum worked or not, Plenck's debut with this intriguing treatise did earn him immediate name recognition.

Plenck wasted no time building his bibliography; in the period between 1767 and 1775, he authored the following works (with titles translated into English), many of which in this first phase of publication covered surgical topics. Several of the works appeared in multiple editions, and almost all of the works on the following list were first published in Latin but later translated into many different languages, including German, French, Italian, Dutch, Spanish, Portuguese, Russian, Lithuanian, and Japanese:

- *A new system of tumors by which these diseases are reduced into their genera and species* (1767)
- *Elements of the art of obstetrics* (1768)

- *Collection of observations on the subject of wound medicine* (1770)
- *Materia chirurgica, or theory of the effects of the remedies used in wound medicine* (1771)
- *Principles of the practice of wound medicine* (1774)
- *Aphorisms for understanding and curing surgical diseases* (1775)
- *Selection of surgical remedies with a list of tools and bandages* (1775)
- *Surgical pharmacy, or the science of prepared and compounded medicinal products* (1775)
- *First line anatomy in practical lessons* (1775)

Doctrina de Morbis Cutaneis was first published in Latin in 1776. That text came during a period in Plenck's publishing career when he was producing many clinical publications.

The texts authored by Plenck in this second phase (1776–1785) are as follows:

- *Instruction on Skin Diseases* (1776)
- *A compendium of surgical institutes for beginners of surgery* (1776)
- *Instruction on diseases of the eye* (1777)
- *Instruction on diseases of the teeth and gums* (1778)
- *Instruction on venereal disease* (1779)
- *Elements of forensic medicine and surgery* (1781)
- *Bromatology, or teachings about foods and drinks* (1785)
- *Toxicology, or teachings on poisons and antidotes* (1785)

The third phase, marking a period in which he was serving at the Josephinum as head of botany and pharmacy, contained the following manuscripts on topics related to his profession:

- *Icons of medicinal plants* (8 volumes published between 1788–1812)
- *Hygrology of the human body, or the chemical-physiological theory of humor contained in the human body* (1794)
- *Physiology and pathology of plants* (1794)
- *The basic principles of botany and the sexual system of plants* (1796)
- *Elements of pharmaco-catagraphs or teaching about medicinal prescription formulas* (1799)
- *Elements of chemistry* (1801)
- *Elements of pharmaceutical chemistry* (1802)
- *Medico-surgical pharmacologia, or instruction on the strength of medicines, mainly used internally and externally in the treatment of diseases* (1804)

In the final phase of his career, Plenck, disabled in body but not in mind, returned to the clinical:

- *Instruction on the diagnosis and treatment of diseases of young children* (1807)
- *Instruction on diseases of the female sex* (published posthumously in 1808)

From the list, it can be seen that Plenck wore many hats during his long career, and he received acclaim in each of the respective fields about which he wrote. His book on obstetrics—his longest work—and his text on venereal disease were particularly noteworthy during his lifetime, reaching a wide audience in the medical schools of Europe. Many of Plenck's texts were succinct handbooks and teaching manuals purposed for instructing medical students on the basics of individual topics in medicine and surgery; as they were commonly used by medical students throughout Europe, they brought him deserved fame during his lifetime. Plenck is recognized as being among the first to recommend that physicians use gloves as they delivered babies born to mothers with syphilis to protect themselves from infection; this was decades before his countryman, Ignaz Semmelweis argued for hand hygiene prior to surgery. Physicians of the eighteenth century commonly showed great interest in botany, and Plenck was no exception. He was an excellent botanist and even has a plant named after him: *Plenckia papulnea*. In sum, Plenck was a highly respected scholar on many different topics, including medicine, surgery, obstetrics, venereology, chemistry, botany, toxicology, pharmacology, ophthalmology, and dentistry.

Plenck's collection of works reached far-away Japan. Fujikawa concluded that Plenck's books were, directly and indirectly, largely responsible for the development of Japanese medicine.[2] The Japanese appreciated the concise and simplistic nature of Plenck's works. His books on surgery, ophthalmology, gynecology, and pediatrics were the first Western works available on these subjects in Japanese.

It is worth noting here that historians of medicine have not placed Plenck very high in their respective pantheons. Heinrich Haeser (1811–1884) called him an "author of an immense number of writings, on all branches of medicine, which are for the most part mediocre." George Fischer noted the bad as well as the good, with his assessment reminding us of Plenck's audience:

> Plenck has no significance as a surgeon and his surgical works are without scientific value. He was, however, an adroit writer who had the gift of getting hold of the kernel of the science in a way which, for the

> most part, was complete and well arranged, even though with somewhat exaggerated brevity. To this circumstance he owes it that his books, especially in Austria, were the favorites for elementary instruction and that they lived through many editions. All his writings were based on the low educational level of the German surgeons.[3]

The author of the first history of dermatology, Paul Richter (1865–1938), wrote:

> Books of the sort indicated, which contain the substance of a whole science demand tireless industry, wide reading and the hand of a master who knows the science in its whole extent and who knows how to distinguish every thing that is essential and to arrange it in order. In the sciences indicated by the titles, I know of no author who has presented the subjects with so complete and well-arranged brevity. He has, besides, utilized everything that recent workers have observed and discovered. From this point of view these books are of value and service not only for beginners but also for the skilled and experienced physician who usually devotes himself to only one branch of his art. For such a one it is pleasant and profitable to cast a glance over the whole field of his science, for, otherwise, with time, many a locality, many a field, into which his practice does not take him, will become unknown and strange.[4]

The Text

Doctrina de Morbis Cutaneis, or "Instruction on Skin Diseases," was first printed in Latin in 1776 and again in 1783 and 1796; in German in 1777 and 1789; in Italian in 1781 and 1785; in Spanish in 1798 and 1816; and in Japanese in 1815. Until now, no English translation has existed. We translated the second Latin edition, published in 1783. The only difference between the second and third edition is that the type-setting is more compact for the third edition, which is a brisk 116 pages; the second edition is 136 pages plus an index. The table of contents provides the Latin and the German name for the disease. It is much shorter than treatises on skin disease that preceded it and followed it, and it is one of the shortest books that Plenck wrote. Its size was ideal for a handbook—a *vade mecum* (literally, "go with me")—a book kept handy by Plenck's audience, who were medical students and inexperienced surgeons expected to care for patients with skin diseases.

The book is dedicated to Giovanni Alessandro Brambilla (1728–1800), an Italian surgeon who served as personal surgeon to Emperor Joseph II. Plenck lauded Brambilla as a most brilliant, expert, learned, and celebrated man.

In the preface, Plenck acknowledged the challenges faced by his students in learning about skin diseases, stemming from "the great number and the diversity of cutaneous diseases, the obscurity of their causes and differences, as well as the difficulty of treating them." He claimed that the study of skin diseases was one of the most difficult and most incomprehensible for his students. As a result, his objective, as stated in the preface, was to "reduce this vast and disparate pile of diseases into a system."

Plenck broke ground with his attempt to distill the known information of his time into a morphology-based system. Contained within the pages of *Doctrina* is a classification system of skin disease that was influenced by Linnaeus and Sauvages and the other nosologists who preceded him. His classification system categorizes 119 skin diseases into 14 categories or "classes." Under each class, Plenck offered "genera" (subtypes of classes) and "species" (subtypes of genera). For example, under the first class, "Maculae," Plenck created 35 different genera of macules, and each of these genera has 3–12 different species. Plenck's use of these descriptive terms for categories of diseases was novel. Dermatologists today still use these terms—macules, papules, pustules, crusts, etc.—to describe the primary skin lesions of a skin disease.

Each disease is given a short description, some as short as one sentence. In contrast to his contemporary Lorry's verbose and flamboyant Latin *Tractatus*, the brevity, conciseness, and clarity of Plenck's entries, in keeping with the handbook length, are the work's greatest attributes and rare for the time. In addition to the descriptions of the physical features of the conditions, Plenck reliably listed treatment options for each condition. Finally, there are footnotes throughout the text containing references to his sources, many of which are contemporary, or brief anecdotes from Plenck's personal experience that supplement the main part of the narrative.

Reception

The reception of *Doctrina* by authorities on skin disease in the generations after Plenck is decidedly mixed. We have found no commentary on *Doctrina* from anyone in Plenck's generation. In the generation that immediately followed Plenck's, a British, skin-minded clinician at the Carey Street Dispensary named Robert Willan, whose morphology-based classification system and revision of the nomenclature earned him the moniker "founder of dermatology," never credited Plenck for his work. Willan's system is much cleaner than Plenck's, and is somewhat more comforting to the modern dermatologist. Willan's protégé, Thomas Bateman (1778–1821), attempted to correct Willan's disregard of Plenck with the following statement:

> It seems probable, indeed, that Dr. Willan was indebted to this work of Professor Plenck for the groundwork of his classification; since his definitions, as well as his terms, accord accurately with those of the Hungarian nosologist.[5]

Perhaps the work's greatest legacy was its utility to Willan. Keizo Dohi (1866–1931) observed that the book "influenced the future great development of dermatology, through its application by Willan, the genius of dermatology."[6]

The French dermatologist Raymond Sabouraud (1864–1938) saw Plenck as the first in a genealogy of founders:

> Just as Plenk [*sic*] begets Willan, and Willan begets Bateman, Bateman, in his turn, begets Biett and the school of the French Willanists. Thus starting with Plenk, the genealogy of the Nineteenth Century dermatologists is clear and without interruption and no break is found.[7]

King and King, writing in the 1980s, wrote the following satisfying assessment of Willan's relationship to Plenck:

> Willan drew heavily from Plenck's dermatologic alphabet, altering and greatly expanding it. Nonetheless, it was Willan who breathed life into the nascent specialty of dermatology, fleshing out the bare bones provided by Plenck 20 years earlier. If Willan is remembered as the father of modern dermatology, Plenck should be recalled as its grandfather.[8]

On the other hand, many of the descendants of Plenck were critical of *Doctrina* in their own writings. One general criticism of the work, as noted by John Lane (1872–1933), was that Plenck had little experience diagnosing and treating the diseases about which he wrote in *Doctrina*. This is unfair because the translation reveals that Plenck frequently wrote "I saw," "I have seen," "I have cured many with," "I discovered that this treatment," and "I have discovered the benefits," indicating a high level of experience with the diseases he addressed. Plenck was also keenly aware of the chaos in dermatological nomenclature as he stated in the preface. Another general criticism of the work, again from Lane, is that it had little staying power and Plenck was able to transmit little of his body of work to subsequent generations. This is fair, but we must remember that the work's intent was to be a small handbook for medical students across Europe. Based on its size alone, it could not compete with the more elaborate works of Lorry, Willan, Jean-Louis Alibert (1768–1837), and Pierre Rayer (1793–1867) in the generations that followed.

A major criticism of the Willanists is that Plenck did not classify the diseases by the primary lesion. Alphee Cazenave (1795–1877) complained that Plenck's diseases went through stages that would put them into multiple classes in his system. For example, Cazenave noted some diseases would start vesicular or pustular and evolve into a crusted or ulcerative stage, and he complained that Plenck listed these diseases in multiple categories (e.g., vesicles and crusts). Pierre Rayer (1793–1867) argued similarly that crusts and ulcers are never primary changes; they always follow pustules, vesicles, bullae, tubercles, and sometimes squamous diseases, and therefore, they should not get their own categories. While these are true statements, they are unfair fault-findings. In *Doctrina*, it is clearly evident that Plenck is aware crusts and ulcers arise from other morphologies. He actually wrote that they did this. His purpose was to teach students what to think about for each morphology. Nowhere in the text does he state that his purpose was to delineate the primary (elemental) lesions. He openly demonstrated in his different sections on crusts and ulcers that the causes are diseases mentioned in other classes.

The appraisal by Moriz Kaposi (1837–1902) of Plenck's contribution is more balanced, but we again must remind ourselves of the fact that Plenck had no intention of categorizing by primary lesion:

> Plenck's *Doctrina de Morbis Cutaneis*, like a catechism, impresses one by its concise and convenient axioms as an apparently sure guide which could not be better adopted for familiarizing one with diseases of the skin. Yet, as soon as these diseases were observed again at the bedside of the patient, it was easy to be convinced that they did not manifest themselves in forms as fixed as the definitions of Plenck indicated, but showed very variable pathologic phenomena and consequently deserved being placed, some in one class, some in another. Thus, an affection which showed papules today, after a little time, appeared in the form of vesicles, and later still under the aspect of bullae, or ulcers. Besides, it is to be regretted that Plenk, confining himself solely to the external form, and not to the essential pathological phenomena, should have joined in the same class processes which were entirely different, like scabies and small pox, acute exanthemata, lenticular macules, leprosy and goose flesh, to say nothing of many pathological monstrosities like syphilitic scabies and other similar things. But the exposition of these precise ideas on the primary lesions of diseases of the skin was nevertheless progress of real value for the future of dermatological studies, in that it suppressed in a definite manner and degree the arbitrariness of the terminology, while facilitating discussion.[9]

In the twentieth century, Gustav Riehl (1855–1943) wrote that Plenck's morphological approach to classification led to a "wholly forced collection of diseases widely differing in their pathology."[10] This is fair, because what is contained within some of the genera is a collection of conditions which have nothing to do with one another. But the conditions share in common the shape of the lesions, and there was little accuracy in understanding of pathology at the time, and not much more in Riehl's era. In addition, this was a student manual, and pathology was not a priority anywhere in the work.

Perhaps it was the aforementioned John Lane who reduced Plenck more than any of the others, while being most complimentary to Willan:

> The chief point of interest is the way in which Plenk became the originator of the modern classification of diseases of the skin. I believe that it was largely—not wholly—a lucky chance. His "De morbis cutaneis" is cast in the same mold as his other books. I imagine that when he sat down to write it, he found that the previous divisions made, those according to the regions of the body, would furnish only a few of the necessary pigeonholes, and that his methodical mind could not contemplate with equanimity the lack of order that would prevail with such a system. And then came the inspiration—the thought that a classification based on the numerous types of lesions would fill the want and make everything orderly. The rest was easy. With the infinite variety of visible manifestations of diseases of the skin, there would be no necessity of leaving any pigeonholes empty, and even the smallest ones he had used in his "Anatomy." He was an admirer and student of Linnaeus, and it is likely that the works of Linnaeus had made him a classifier.
>
> The idea of using the anatomic lesions as the basis of the classification was a brilliant one for which Plenk should have due credit. But that is all the credit that can be claimed for him in that line, for a great dermatologist he was not. Aside from the method of classification, there is not a new idea in his book, and his observation—if indeed the book was chiefly based on observation—was not superior to that of his predecessors. Willan, the keen observer, careful student, trained physician and brilliant dermatologist, saw the use that could be made of the classification, modified it, adopted it, and kept it alive.[11]

These men seemed to go out of their way both to forget Plenck's purpose and to find fault with Plenck's ingenious and mold-breaking accomplishment. It is not impossible to conclude that the nineteenth-century medical men—caught up in the passions of being the forerunners of a budding specialty in places like London, Paris, and even Plenck's hometown of Vienna—purposefully downplayed Plenck's contribution in order to elevate their own, especially in the case of Robert Willan. It is our contention that the "Cult of Willan" (coined by Alan Lyell) led by the French "Willanistes" of the 1820s and 1830s, such as Cazenave, could not risk their man's legacy being upstaged by a relatively obscure Hungarian surgeon from the 1770s. Thus, the impact of Plenck's contribution ultimately ended without fanfare when his life ended, especially because Plenck had no Thomas Bateman as Robert Willan did, or no Laurent Biett as Jean-Louis Alibert did, or no Moriz Kaposi as Ferdinand von Hebra did to carry on his work and amplify his legacy. Moreover, Plenck was a polymath, and polymaths in the history of dermatology—even genius ones such as Jonathan Hutchinson—do not get the same credit as individuals who focused all of their energies on the skin alone. Perhaps access in the English language to Plenck's important text will increase the credit long owed to Joseph Jacob Plenck.

Notes About the Translation

The authors would like to point out several aspects of the translation and its formatting. Any word that is underlined in the translation has an entry in the glossary in the back of the book, because dermatologists still use Latin diagnostic terms today, we retained these terms for the headings in the English translation, but a translation of these diagnoses can be found in brackets adjacent to the heading. In the rare instance that there is no translation of the Latin term, a discussion can be found under the glossary entry for the term. All italicized words in the English translation were italicized by Plenck in his Latin. Finally, Plenck's footnotes were moved to the end of the chapters as endnotes, and all endnotes in the translation are Plenck's, not the authors'. All author commentary on the translation can be found in the glossary.

References

1 Lane, J.E. Joseph Jacob Plenk 1738?–1807. Arch Derm Syphilol. 1933;28(2):193–214.
2 ibid.
3 ibid.
4 ibid.
5 Bateman, T. Practice Synopsis of Cutaneous Diseases. London: Longman, Hurst, Rees, Orme, and Brown, 1814. p. xi.
6 Lane, J.E. Joseph Jacob Plenk 1738?–1807. Arch Derm Syphilol. 1933;28(2):193–214.
7 ibid.
8 King, D.F., and King, L.A. Josef Plenck–Grandfather of Modern Dermatology. J Am Acad Dermatol. 1984;11(1):143–6.
9 Lane, J.E. Joseph Jacob Plenk 1738?–1807. Arch Derm Syphilol. 1933;28(2):193–214.
10 ibid.
11 ibid.

Translation

JOSEPHI JACOBI PLENCK

Chirurgiae Doctoris, nec non Chirurgiae, Anatomes atque Artis Obstetriciae Professoris Regii, publici ac ordinarii in Regia Universitate Budensi.

Doctrina

de

Morbis Cutaneis

Qua Hi Morbi in Suas Classes, Genera et Species Rediguntur.

Editio Secunda, aucta.

Viennae,

Apud Rudolphum Graeffer.

1783.

JOSEPH JACOB PLENCK

Surgical Doctor, not only of Surgery and Anatomy, but also Royal Professor of the Art of Obstetrics, publicus ordinarius in the Royal University of Buda.

Instruction

on

Cutaneous Diseases

In which these Diseases are Ordered into their own Classes, Genera, and Species.

Second Edition, augmented

Vienna

Published by Rudolph Graeffer

1783

Viro
Perillustri, expertissimo,
Doctissimo, ac Celeberrimo
Joanni Alexandro Brambilla
Sac. Caes. Reg. Apost. Maj.
Chirurgo Primario
nec non
Exercituum et Praetorianorum imperialium chirurgo supremo
Academiae Chirurgicae regiae parisiensis, montispesul. Bononiensis et mantinens. Membro
Hoc qualecunque opusculum in amicitiae, observantiaeque monumentum
Dedicat et Consecrat

Author.

The author dedicates and consecrates this little work, of whatever quality it may be, as a memorial to friendship and in deference to the most illustrious, most experienced, most learned and most celebrated man, Joanni Alexandro Brambilla (Sac. Caes. Reg. Apost. Maj.), Chief Surgeon, also Supreme Surgeon of the Imperial Army and Praetorians, Member of the Royal Surgical Academy of Paris, Montepellier, Bologna, and Mantua.

PRAEFATIO

Morborum, qui cutem humanam affligunt, multitudo, atque varietas, caussarum, a quibus, ii proveniunt, obscuritas, & quae inde nascitur sanandi difficultas, diversitasque, hanc medicinae, chirurgiaeque doctrinam tyronibus difficillimam & vix extricabilem reddidere. Authores demum, quos consultum adire licet, pauci sunt, quorum alii hoc, licet omnis aevi frequens morborum genus, nonnisi citissimo tetigere calamo; alii vago ac non constanti nominum usu diagnosim, curandique rationem effecere incertam.

Haec sunt, quae me incitabant, ut hanc vastam indigestamque horum morborum molem in systema redigere adlaborarem. Opusculum hoc, quod in usum meorum Auditorum concinnaveram, centum & quindecim genera complectitur affectuum cutaneorum; morbos chronicos diligenter descripsi, exanthematum autem febrilium solam adjeci differentiam & diagnosim, qua a se & a similibus distinguantur; curatio enim exanthematum febrilium in sola sanatione febris, a qua profluunt, consistit, quae ad aliam pathologiae spartam pertinet.

Multum equidem, gratus fateor, celeberrimis viris, qui nuper generica morborum systemata condidere, **Sauvagesio, Linnaeo, Vogelio, Macbridio, Cullenio, Sagaro, Hartmanno, Lorryo, Danielio**, debeo, quorum systematibus saepe cum uberrimo fructu ufus sum nec tamen superfluam me navasse operam opinor, si ea attendas, quae adjeci, correxi, dilucidavi.

PREFACE

The great number of diseases that afflict the human skin, as well as their variety, the obscurity of the causes from which they come forth, and the difficulty and diversity of healing what is produced by them, have rendered this branch of medicine and of surgery the most difficult and scarcely comprehensible for those initiating in medicine. The authors whom we are able to consult up until this point are few, some of whom describe the kind of diseases common to every age, unless they were touched by very swift divine intervention; others use vague and inconsistent diagnostic names, and they formulate an uncertain reason for the cure.

These are the things that have spurred me to labor to reduce this vast and disparate pile of diseases into a system. This little work, which I had prepared for the use of my pupils, includes 115 kinds of conditions of the skin. I have diligently described chronic diseases, but in addition I specifically concentrated on the differential diagnosis of febrile exanthems, which are distinguished from one another and from similar diseases. Indeed the treatment of febrile exanthems merely consists of quieting the fever from which they flow, which pertains to another sphere of pathology.

Certainly I am most grateful for the very celebrated men who recently founded systems of general diseases; I am indebted to Sauvages, Linnaeus, Vogel, Macbride, Cullen, Sagar, Hartmann, Lorry, and Daniel, whose systems I used often with very productive results. However I do not think—if you attend to it—that I have done a superfluous work, to which I have directed my mind, corrected, and elucidated.

CLASSES MORBORUM CUTANEORUM

I. Maculae, die Flecke.
II. Pustulae, die Eiterblattern.
III. Vesiculae, die Wasserblattern.
IV. Bullae, die Blasen.
IV. Papulae, die Knoten.
V. Crustae, die Rauden.
VI. Squammae, die Schuppen.
VII. Callositates, die Schwüllen.
IX. Excrescentiae cutanea, die Hautgewächse.
X. Ulcera cutanea, die Hautgeschwüre.
XI. Vulnera cutanea, die Hautwunden.
XII. Insecta cutanea, die Hautinfekten.
XIII. Morbi unguium, die Nägelkrankheiten.
XIV. Morbi pilorum, die Haarkrankheiten.

CLASSES OF CUTANEOUS DISEASES

I. Macules
II. Pustules
III. Vesicles
IV. Bullae
V. Papules
VI. Crusts
VII. Scales
VIII. Calluses
IX. Cutaneous Growths
X. Cutaneous Ulcers
XI. Cutaneous Wounds
XII. Cutaneous Insects
XIII. Diseases of the Nail
XIV. Diseases of the Hair

GENERA ET SPECIES MORBORUM CUTANEORUM.

Classis I. Maculae.

Maculae fuscae.

Lentigo, *die Sommersprosse.*
Ephelis, *die Leberflecke.*
Fuscedo cutis, *die braune Haut.*
Flavedo cutis, *die gelbe Haut.*

Macula rubra.

Gutta rosacea, *der Kupferbandel.*
Stigma, *der rothe Punkt.*
Erythema, *die Hautröthe.*
Morbilli, *die Kindsflecken.*
Scarlatina, *der Scharlachausschlag.*
Urticaria, *der Brennesselausschlag.*
Maculae venereae, *die venerische Flecke.*
Esserae, *die flache rothe Flecke.*
Psydraciae, *die erhobene rothe Flecke.*
Rubedo cutis, *die rothe Haut.*
Zona seu Zoster, *die Feuergürtel.*
Macula lata Plateri, seu Ignis sacer, *der Feuerflecke*

Maculae lividae.

Ecchymoma, *der blaue Flecke.*
Livor cutis, *die Schwarzblaue Haut.*
Vibex, *der Streif.*
Maculae scorbuticae, *die Scharbocksflecke.*
Maculae gangraenosae, *die Brandflecke.*
Petechiae, *die Fetechen.*

GENERA AND SPECIES OF CUTANEOUS DISEASES

Class I. Macules

Dark Macules

Lentigo
Freckle
Dark skin
Yellow skin

Red Macules

Rosacea
Marks
Erythema
Measles
Scarlet fever
Febrile urticaria
Venereal spots
Non-febrile urticaria
Vesiculobullous lesions
Red skin
Herpes zoster (shingles)
Erysipelas

Livid spots

Bruised spots
Bruised areas
Linear bruise
Scurvy spots
Gangrenous spots
Petechiae

Maculae nigrae.

Melas, *der Schwarzgefleckte Aussatz.*
Melasma, *der Schwarze Flecke.*
Noma, *der Kinderbrand, oder Todtenwurm.*
Nigredo cutis, *die Schwarze Haut.*

Maculae albae.

Alphos, *der weisgefleckte Ausfatz.*
Albor cutis, *die weisse Haut.*
Pallor cutis, *die bleiche Haut*

Maculae incerti coloris.

Maculae maternae, *die Muttermahle.*
Maculae artificiales, *die gekünstelte Flecke.*
Cutis variegata, *die gefleckte Haut.*
Cutis fucata, *die geschminkte Haut.*
Cutis unctuosa, *die glänzende Haut.*

Classis II. Pustulae.

Pustulae, *die Eiterfinnen.*
Scabies, *die Krätze.*
Variolae, *die Kindspocken.*
Varicellae, *die unächten Kindspocken.*
Terminthus, *die Erbsenblattern.*

Classis III. Vesiculae.

Sudamen, *die Schweisblattern.*
Miliare, *die Friselblattern.*
Hydatis, *die Wasserblasen.*
Vesiculae cristallinae genitalium, *die Crystalblattern der Schaamtheilen.*
Uritis, *die Brennblattern.*

Classis IV. Bullae.

Phyma, *die Eiterblasen.*
Bullae, *die Wasserblasen.*
Pemphygus, *der Blasenausschlag.*

Black spots

Black morphea/black vitiligo
Melasma
Noma
Blackened skin

White spots

Vitiligo
White skin
Pale skin

Spots of Uncertain Color

Birthmarks
Artificial spots
Variegated skin
Painted skin
Oily skin

Class II. Pustules

Pustules
Scabies
Smallpox
Chickenpox
Folliculitis

Class III. Vesicles

Afebrile miliaria
Febrile miliaria
Hidrocystoma
Genital vesicles
Nocturnal and diurnal vesicles

Class IV. Bullae

Abscess
Bullae
Pemphigus/pemphigoid

Classis V. Papulae.

Vari, *die Finnen.*
Grutum, *der Gries.*
Herpes seu Serpigo, *die Flechte.*
Cutis anserina, *die Gänshaut.*
Tuberculum, *der Knote.*
Phygethlon, *die rothe Knoten.*
Lepra, *der Aussatz*
Elephantiasis, *der Elefantenaussatz.*

Classis VI. Crustae.

Crusta, *die Raude.*
Eschara, *der Schorf.*
Achores, *die Kopfraude.*
Crusta capitis neunatorum, *der Kneis.*
Crusta lactea, *der Milchgrind.*
Tinea, *der Grind.*
Mentagra, *der Kieferaussatz.*
Malum mortuum, *das todte Uebel.*
Exanthema labiale, *der Lippenausschlag.*
Exanthema subaxillare, *der Achfelhöhlausfchlag.*

Classis VII. Squammae.

Furfuratio, *die Hautkleien.*
Desquammatio, *das Abschuppen der Haut.*
Exuvia epidermidis, *der Abgang der Oberhaut.*
Porrigo, *der Kleiengrind.*
Lichen, *der Zitterich.*
Impetigo, *der Kleienaussatz.*
Ichthyosis, *der Fischschuppenaussatz.*
Tyriasis, *der Schlangenaussat.*
Asperitas cutis, *die Rauhigkeit der Haut.*
Rugositas cutis, *die Runzeln der Haut.*

Classis VIII. Callositates.

Callus, *die Schwülle.*
Cicatrix, *die Maser.*
Clavus, *das Hüneraug.*

Class V. Papules

Acne
Milia
Herpes
Goosebumps
Nodules
Abscess
Lepra
Hansen's disease

Class VI. Crusts

Crusts
Eschars
Tinea capitis
Cradle cap
Facial eczema
Tinea
Impetigo
Dead evil
Herpes labialis
Bullous impetigo

Class VII. Scales

Dandruff
Desquamation
Exfoliation
Seborrheic dermatitis
Lichen
Psoriaisis
Ichthyosis
Tyriasis
Rough skin
Wrinkled skin

Class VIII. Calluses

Calluses
Scar
Corns

Classis IX. Excrescentiae Cutaneae

Verruca, *die Warze.*
Cornua, *die Hauthörner.*
Hystricismus, *der Stachelaussat*
Condyloma, *die Feigwang.*
Frambaesia, *der Schwammformig Aussatz.*

Classis X. Ulcera Cutanea

Excoriatio purulenta, *die Hautschwürung.*
Intertrigo, *der Frat.*
Aphthae, *die Mundschwämchen.*
Fissurae, *das Hautaufspringen.*
Rhagades, *die Hautschrunden.*

Classis XI. Vulnera Cutanea

Excoriatio cruenta, *die Hautaufschärfung.*
Scissura, *der Schnitt.*
Pressura, *der Zwicker.*
Morsus, *der Bis.*
Punctura, *der Stich.*
Ictus ab insecto, *der Insekten Stich.*

Classis XII. Insecta Cutanea.

Phthiriasis, *die Laussucht.*
Helmintiasis, *die Hautwurmsucht.*
Malis, *die Insektengeschwülste.*
Crinones, *die Mitesser.*

Classis XIII. Morbi Unguium.

Seline, *der weisse Nagelflecke.*
Ecchymoma, *der blaue Nagelflecke.*
Gryphosis, *die Nagelkrümmung.*
Fissura unguium, *der Nagelspalt.*
Tinea unguium, *der Nagelgrind.*
Mollities unguium, *die Weichheit der Nägel.*
Scabrities unguium, *die Hokerigkeit der Nägel.*

Class IX. Cutaneous Growths

Warts
Horns
Ichthyosis hystrix
Condyloma
Yaws

Class X. Cutaneous Ulcers

Excoriation
Intertrigo
Aphthosis
Fissures
Rhagades

Class XI. Cutaneous Wounds

Scratch
Laceration
Pinch
Bite
Puncture
Insect bite

Class XII. Cutaneous Insects

Lice
Worms
Bug bites
Crinones

Class XIII. Diseases of the Nail

Leukonychia
Bruised nails
Onychogryphosis
Fissured nail
Tinea unguium
Soft nails
Dry nails

Pterigium unguis, *das Nagelfell.*
Arctura unguis, *der Nagelzwang, das Nagelshwür.*
Deformitas unguis, *die Ungestaltheit der Nägel.*
Lapsus unguis, *der Abfall der Nägel.*

Classis XIV. Morbi Pilorum.

Calvities, *der Kahlkopf.*
Hirsuties, *die Haarigkeit.*
Xerasia, *die Dünhaarigkeit.*
Trichoma, *der Wichtelzopf.*
Fissuras capillorum, *die gespaltete Haare.*
Canities, *der Graukopf.*

Pterygium unguis
Ingrown nail
Deformed nail
Shedding of nail

Class XIV. Diseases of the Hair

Hair loss
Excessive hair
Thin hair
Plicated hair
Split hair
Gray hair

DE MORBIS CUTANEIS GENERATIM

Morbi, qui cutem ejusque partes infestant, *cutanei* vocantur.

Hi dividi solent

1. in *acutos*, quic um febre erumpunt, & cum illa evanescunt
2. in *chronicos*, qui sine febresunt & utplurimum diu durare affuescunt.

Ast facilioris intellectus gratia omnes morbos cutaneos in sequentes, a morbi indole petitas, XIV divido classes.

ON CUTANEOUS DISEASES BY CATEGORIES

Diseases, which affect the skin and its parts, are called *cutaneous*.

These are commonly divided into:

1. *acute*, which erupt with fever, and vanish as the fever resolves.
2. *chronic*, which are without fever and usually last, for the most part, a very long time.

But for the sake of easier understanding, I divide all cutaneous diseases that follow, based on the nature of the disease, into 14 classes.

CLASSIS I. MACULAE

Sunt locales coloris nativi mutationes in cute.

Sedes materiae morbosae intra cutem & epidermidem in reticulo celluloso epidermidis est.

Color macularum est varius, ruber, fuscus, lividus, niger, albus.

Demum hae maculae, vel *solitariae*, vel *agminatae* erumpunt.

Curatio pro materiae morbosae diversita diversa est.

Species macularum sunt sequentes.

Lentigines

Sunt maculae fusca, quae colore, figura & magnitudine lentes referunt.

Partes soli expositae, ut facies, dorsa manuum, rarius antica crurum superficies, his maculis affici solent.

Puellas albidas cum ruffis capillis maxim aggreditur lentigo. Aestate augentur, & hiema descrescunt hae maculae.

Cum autem lentigo in partibus non insolatis etiam oriatur, & at moniales, soli non expositas, etiam afficiat, atque ulcera in lentiginosis cacoetha saepe evadant, hinc peculiaris cacochymia *causa* lentiginis esse videtur.

Curatio. Cum specificum cacochymiae lentiginosae remedium adhuc ignoretur, hinc depurantia generalia *interne* adhibeantur. Serum lactis tamarindinatum & juscula ex chaerophyllo & aliis herbis hepaticis, utilia deprehendi.

Externe acetum armoraciae,[1] fel taurinum,[2] pasta amygdalarum amararum, lac sulphuris, aqua phagaedenica, & solutio vitrioli albi laudatur.

[1] Cel. Kruniz *oeconomische Encyclopedie* 2. Vol. pag. 127.

CLASS I. MACULES

Macules are local changes in the native color of the skin.

The seat of morbid material within the skin and epidermis is in the cellular network of the epidermis.

The color of macules is various: red, dark, livid, black, white.

Finally, these spots erupt, either as *solitary* or *grouped.*

Treatment differs due to the diversity of the morbid material.

The species of macules are the following:

Lentigines [sun spots/age spots]

Lentigines are dark spots that look like lentils in color, shape, and size.

The parts exposed to the sun—the face, back of the hands, and more rarely the front surface of the legs—are commonly affected by these macules.

Lentigo mostly affects white women with red hair. In the summer, these macules increase, and they diminish in the winter.

However, a malignant ulcer often arises in lentigines on parts protected from the sun, even affecting nuns not exposed to the sun; hence, the cause of this particular lentigo seems to be a bad humor.

Treatment. Since the specific remedy for the bad humor of lentigo is as yet unknown, at this point general cleansings internally may be employed. I have discovered the benefits of tamarind whey and juice of chervil and other hepatic herbs.

Externally, the vinegar of horseradish,[1] the bile of oxen,[2] the paste of bitter almonds, the milk of sulfur, phagedenic water, and solution of white vitriol are recommended.

[1] Celebrated Kruniz' *Oeconomicsche Encyclopedia* vol 2 p. 127.

[2] Cel. Geoffroi in *Memoires de 'Academ. de Scienc.* adversus lenticulas seu lentigines faciei cosmeticum ex felle tauri, oleo tartari per deliquium & aqua, laudat. Cel. Hartmannus p. 794. ex bile cosmeticum parat, de quo dicit: *ad miraculum usque albedinem cuti conciliat.*

Ephelis

Est macula fusca, lata, solitaria vel agminata.

Species ephelidum sunt:

1. **Ephelis solaris**, quae in facie & manu ab insolatione in teneris puellis observatur. *Praecavetur* umbraculis, pileo magno, chirothecis.

Curatur lavatorio ex oxycrato, aqua camphorata, petrosellino in aqua frigida macerato, pasta amygdalarum.

2. **Ephelis ignealis**. Post cutis ambustionem remanet, etiam in feminarum tibiis & femoribus observatur, quae hyeme foculos pedibus supponunt. Etiam a vesicatorio, si cuticola aufertur, saepe fusca & lata macula diu remanet.

Curatio a tempore exspectanda.

3. **Ephelis gravidarum**. Maculae fuscae, solitariae, palmam latae, frontem praecipue afficientes, in gravidis observantur, quas *maculas gravidarum* vocant.

Hae maculae post partum evanescunt.

4. **Ephelis hepatica**. In virginibus difficulter menstruantibus, & quandoque in viris haemorrhoide caeca laborantibus, & in aliis, quibus hepar afficitur, observantur hae maculae, quas etiam *Hepatizon* dicunt.

Curatio exigit, ut fluxus retentus restituatur. Externe applicantur, quae in lentigine & ephelide solari laudantur.

[2] Celebrated Geoffery in *Memoirs of the Academy of Science*, praises a cosmetic use against lentils or lentigines of the face that is made from ox bile, oil of tartar per deliquium, and water. The Celebrated Hartmann prepares a cosmetic from bile about which he says, "it marvelously and completely restores the whiteness of the skin."

Ephelis [freckles]

Ephelis is a dark, broad spot, solitary or grouped.

The species of freckles are:

1. **Ephelis solaris** [freckle from sun, sun spot] is observed on the face and hand after sun exposure in young girls. It is prevented with parasols, a large cap, and gloves.

It is treated with oxycrate bath, camphor water, parsley soaked in cold water, almond paste.

2. **Ephelis ignealis** [freckle from fire, erythema ab igne] remains after a burn of the skin, observed likewise on the shins and thighs of women, who stand by the hearth in the winter. Even if the skin is removed by a blistering agent, the dark and broad spot often remains for a long time.

The cure is to wait for it to resolve over time.

3. **Ephelis gravidarum** [freckle of pregnancy, melasma]. Dark, solitary spots, broad as a palm, are observed in pregnant women, especially affecting the forehead, which they call *maculas gravidarum* (spots of pregnancy).

These spots vanish postpartum.

4. **Ephelis hepatica** [liver spot, lentigo]. In virgins with difficult menstruation, and sometimes in men laboring with an internal hemorrhoid, and in others whose liver is impaired, these macules are observed which they even say are *liver-colored.*

Treatment requires that the halted flow be restored. Those things that are recommended for lentigines and solar ephelids are applied externally.

5. **Ephelis neunatorum**. Est macula lutea, quae hinc inde in infantibus neonatis observatur. *Curatur* ut icterus.

Fuscedo Cutis

Est fuscedo non maculosa, sed diffusa per faciem, manus, vel totum corpus.

Species fuscedinis sunt:

1. **Fuscedo aetatis**. Albedo infantum intra aliquot menses in subluteum vel subflavum colorem abit. Viris plerisque, senibus autem omnibus cutis fusca fit.

2. **Fuscedo solaris**. Solis ardor in saturando corporis colore magnam vim habet. Europeis candidis pars frontis pileo tecta, aut pars brachii, vestibus contenta, a reliqua nuda facie nudaque manu distat. Milites multa experti, & peregrinatores, qui calidissimas regiones frequentarunt, e terris remotis faciem fuscam vel atram referunt, quam successive in patria iterum amittunt. At feminae in Asia, gynaecaeis reclusae, manent albae. In climate calidissimo fusci sunt europaei, & in Europa aethiopes aliquantum albidiores fiunt.

Curatio fuscedinis a remediis *cosmeticis* exspectari, rarissime obtineri potest.

3. **Fuscedo nativa**. Aethiops cum albo homine mulattos flavos gignit, qui etiam prodeunt, si mulatti cum mulattis rem habeant. Si vero mulatti cum albo coiverunt, foetus prodit europaeo propior, & post quartam generationem homo ab europaeo non diversus. Si vero cum aethiope rem habeant mulatti, aethiopi propior generatur proles, & post quartam generationem verus redit aethiops. Demum in multis europaeis feminis regio pubis & areolae mammarum fusca, subinde nigricantes sunt.

5. **Ephelis neonatorum** [freckle of the newborn / neonatal jaundice]. It is a yellow spot that is observed at random on a neonatal infant. It is treated the same as jaundice.

Fuscedo Cutis [dark skin]

Fuscedo cutis is dark skin not in spots, but diffusely over the face, hands, or the entire body.

The species of fuscedo are:

1. **Fuscedo aetatis** [dark skin of the aged, photoaging]. The whiteness of infants changes to a yellowish or blondish color within a few months. In very many men, but in all of the elderly, the skin becomes dark.

2. **Fuscedo solaris** [dark skin from the sun, tanning]. The heat of the sun has great strength in saturating the body with color. For white Europeans, the part of the forehead covered with a cap, or the part of the arm covered by their clothes, is distinct from the rest of their naked face and hand. Many experienced soldiers and travelers, who frequent the hottest regions, return from remote countries with a dark or black face, which they subsequently lose again in their own country. But women in Asia, cloistered in women's quarters, remain white. In the hottest climate, the Europeans are dark, and in Europe, the Ethiopians become somewhat whiter.

The treatment of fuscedo, expected from cosmetic remedies, is very rarely able to be obtained.

3. **Fuscedo nativa** [native dark skin]. An Ethiopian woman with a white man gives birth to light-skinned mulattos. If the mulattos have relations with each other, the resulting offspring are also mulattos. If indeed the mulattos have relations with a white person, the fetus produced is closer to European, and after the fourth generation, the person does not differ from a European. But if the mulattos have relations with an Ethiopian, the offspring produced is closer to Ethiopian, and after the fourth generation, a true Ethiopian returns. Finally, in many European women, the pubic region and the areolae of the breasts are brown, and occasionally blackish.

Flavedo Cutis

Est cutis flavedo in tota facie vel toto corpore.

1. **Flavedo icteritia ab ictero seu bile**, in sanguinem redeunte, pender. V. *Icterus.*

2. **Flavedo a sugillatione**. Ecchymosis livida, quamprimum resolvi incipit, flavescit; solitarii enim globuli sanguinis, multo sero diluti, flavescunt.

3. **Flavedo nativa**. In mediterraneis Aethiopiae locis flavae sunt gentes integre.

Gutta Rosacea

Est corymbus macularum rubrarum in facie & naso.

Species guttae rosaceae sunt:

1. **Gutta rosacea simplex** est rubedo nasi & partium adjacentium absque omni asperitate, efflorescentia, pruritu, & desquammatione, diu permanens.

Curatur purgantibus.

2. **Gutta rosacea oenopotarum seu Bacchia**. Format maculas rubras, aliquantum elevatas, & furfuraceas, vini potatoribus est familiaris, & nasum eorum tuberosum reddit. Quandoque brachia, collum & pectus occupat.

Curatio est difficillima, et exigit abstinentiam a vino. Absorbentia, herbae alcalescentes, aqua selterana, juscula millepedum, viperarum, cancrorum, testudinum, succi antiscorbutici, praesertim fumariae, cum purgantibus adhibeantur.

Externe aqua vegetomineralis cum felle taurino: petrosellinum maceratum, aqua phagaedenica tentari potest. Sed cave ne acrimonia repellatur.

3. **Gutta rosacea hydropotarum**. Plures curavi suadendo, ut vinum bibere incipiant.

Flavedo Cutis [yellow skin]

Flavedo cutis is yellow skin on the entire face or the entire body.

1. **Flavedo icteritia** [jaundice] is due to jaundice or bile returning to the blood. See *Icterus.*

2. **Flavedo a sugillatione** [yellow skin from bruising]. The livid ecchymosis, as soon as it begins to be resolved, turns yellow; indeed, the individual blood cells, diluted in so much serum, turn yellow.

3. **Flavedo nativa** [native yellow skin]. In the central parts of Ethiopia, there are races of fully yellow people.

Gutta Rosacea [rosacea]

Gutta rosacea is a cluster of red spots on the face and nose.

The species of gutta rosacea are:

1. **Gutta rosacea simplex** [simple rosacea] is a redness of the nose and the adjacent parts, without any roughness, swelling, itching, or scaling, lasting for a long time.

It is cured with purges.

2. **Gutta rosacea oenopotarum seu Bacchia** [rosacea of the wine-drinker or Bacchia rosacea]. It forms red spots, somewhat elevated and finely scaled, familiar to wine drinkers, and it renders their nose tuberous. Sometimes it affects the arms, neck, and chest.

The treatment is most difficult and requires abstinence from wine. De-acidifying absorbents, slightly alkaline herbs, seltzer water, broth of millipede, vipers, crabs, tortoises, antiscorbutic juices, especially *Fumaria*, are to be used with purges.

Externally, aqua vegetomineralis with bull's gall: soaked parsley, phagedenic water, can be tried. But beware that the impurity is not driven back into the body.

3. **Gutta rosacea hydropotarum** [rosacea of water drinkers]. I have cured very many by persuading them to begin to drink wine.

4. **Gutta rosacea febrilis**. Si in febribus malignis nasus purpureas, bruneus, nigricans, tumidus, pustulosus, evadit, mors instar, ex 20 vix 2 evadunt.[1]

5. **Gutta rosacea pernionalis**. Rubor chronicus nasi a gelu. *Curatur* unguento ad perniones.

6. **Gutta rosacea herpetica**. Est pruriens, vesiculosa & furfurascens.

Curatur ut herpes.

7. **Gutta rosacea syphilitica**. Signa luis venereae habet. Vide *maculas venereas*.

8. **Gutta rosacea lactentium**. In lactentibus maculae rubrae circa genas & labia oriuntur, in cuius centro foramen fuscum & siccum apparet. Hae maculae diu permanent, aliquando in crustam lacteam abeunt, at non semper. Curatio exigit decoctum violae tricoloris. V. *Crusta lactea*.

9. **Gutta rosacea variolosa**. Maculae rubrae in genis post variolas toleratas saepe per medium annum remanent. Evanescunt suasponte. Sed citius, si oleum been cuti illinatur.[2]

[1] De. Meyserey T. 2. n. 241.
[2] Cel. Bruckmann *diss. de nuce Been, Helmst.* 1750. p. 27. memorabilia hujus rei exempla recenset.

Stigma

Est punctum coloris coccinei, in facie vel alia parte. Species sunt:

1. **Stigmata nativa** incurabilia sunt.

2. **Stigmata rubra**, quae subinde subito in facie a violenta *tussi* vel *vomitu* oriuntur, suasponte evanescunt, sic etiam a *scorbuto*, a suppressis

4. **Gutta rosacea febrilis** [febrile rosacea]. If in a malignant fever, the nose becomes purple, brownish, blackened, swollen, or pustular, the equivalent of death ensues; out of 20, barely two recover.[1]

5. **Gutta rosacea pernionalis** [rosacea of pernio]. Chronic red nose from the cold. It is treated with the ointment for pernio (chilblains).

6. **Gutta rosacea herpetica** [herpetic rosacea] is itchy, vesicular, and finely scaled.

It is treated as herpes.

7. **Gutta rosacea syphilitica** [syphilitic rosacea] is a sign the patient has venereal disease. See *venereal macules.*

8. **Gutta rosacea lactentium** [rosacea of the suckling infant]. In suckling infants, red spots arise around the cheeks and lips, in the center of which a dusky and dry opening appears. These spots remain for a long time; sometimes, they evolve into *crusta lactea* (milky crust), but not always. The treatment requires a decoction of the wild pansy. See *crusta lactea.*

9. **Gutta rosacea variolosa** [rosacea from smallpox]. Red spots on the cheeks often last half a year after tolerated smallpox. They fade spontaneously. But sooner, if oil of behen-nut is smeared on the skin.[2]

[1]Guillaume Mahieu de Meyserey. *La Medecine d'armée.* France: Cavelier, 1754. Book II, n. 241.
[2] Urban Friedrich Benedict Bruckman. *Dissertation on the Behen nut.* Helmstadium, 1750. p. 27. He recounts memorable examples of this subject.

Stigma [marks]

Stigma is a pinpoint of scarlet color on the face or other parts. The species are:

1. **Stigmata nativa** [birthmarks] are incurable.

2. **Stigmata rubra** [red marks, petechiae], which on occasion suddenly arise on the face after a violent *cough* or *emesis,* spontaneously fade; such

menstruis, talia rubra stigmata in toto corpore vel in una solummodo parte observantur.

Curatio exigit ut morbus, cuius haec stigmata symptoma sunt, curetur.

3. **Stigmata nigra** a pulvere, pyrio in faciem exploso, exigunt, ut granula pulveris dentiscalpio eximantur.

Erythema

Est cutis macula rubra, solitaria, apyreta & topica, non ut erysipelas per totam partem diffusa. Species sunt:

1. **Erythema ab igne**. Macula rubra, igne inducta, optime curatur, si ardor aqua frigida sopiatur, & dein aqua alba vel unguentum plumbatum applicetur.

2. **Erythema a gelu**. Est rubor cum levi tumore glabro & splendente, ad mutationem aeris hyeme pruriens. Nasum, digitos manuum & pedum atque calcaneos afficit. Frigus extrahitur nive vel aqua frigida, rubor curatur unguento ad perniones.

3. **Erythema ab attritu**. Rubedo clunium in equitantibus, rubedo manuum in operariis & pedum in peditibus huc pertinet.

Curatur applicato sevo recenti, butyro cacao aut unguento plumbato.

4. **Erythema a decubitu**. In regione coccygis & ossis sacri vel illi aegrotum, diu decumbentium, observatur. *Curatio* exigit corium molle & pulvinaria excavata, quibus lumbi & femora sustineantur, ne coccyx a lecto prematur; rubor loci Aqua Thediana,[1] unguento plumbato vel linimento ex albumine & spiritu vini tegatur. Idem fiat, si sub sanatione fracturae cruris a decubitu erythema in calcaneo pedis, oriatur.

red spots are also observed on the whole body or only one part of the body from *scurvy* and from suppressed *menstruation*.

The treatment requires that the disease, of which these spots are symptoms, be cured.

3. **Stigmata nigra** [black marks, gunpowder marks], from the dust when gunpowder explodes in the face, require that the powdery granules be extracted with a toothpick.

Erythema

Erythema is a solitary, red spot of skin, non-feverish and superficial, not spread throughout the entire area as in erysipelas. The species are:

1. **Erythema ab igne** [erythema from fire]. A red spot, induced by fire, is best treated if the burning is soothed with cold water, and then aqua alba or lead ointment is applied.

2. **Erythema a gelu** [erythema from the cold]. It is a redness with a slight swelling, smooth and glistening, and itching due to change in the air during winter. It affects the nose, the digits of the hands and feet, and even the heels. The coldness is drawn out with snow or cold water; the redness is treated with the ointment for chilblains.

3. **Erythema ab atrittu** [erythema from wear and tear, friction burn]. This pertains to the redness of the buttocks in those who ride horses, the redness of the hands of laborers, and the feet of foot travelers.

It is treated with the application of fresh tallow, cocoa butter, or lead ointment.

4. **Erythema a decubitu** [erythema from lying in bed, bedsore]. It is observed in the region of the coccyx and sacrum, in those of the sick, lying in a bed for a long time. Treatment requires soft hide and hollow cushions, on which the loins and thighs should be supported, so that the coccyx is not pressed against the bed; the redness of the place should be covered with Thedian water,[1] lead ointment or liniment of albumen, and with spirits of wine (alcohol). The same may be done if, during the healing of a fracture of the leg, erythema arises on the heel of the foot from lying in bed.

5. **Erythema ab ictu insecti**. Praesentissimum remedium est applicatio aquae frigidae vel petrosellini in aqua macerati.

6. **Erythema ab applicatis acribus**, ut vesicatorio, synapismo, urica.

Curatur butyro non salito.

7. **Erythema volaticum genarum** est subitanous rubor genarum & faciei, qui brevi iterum evanescit. Observatur in verminosis, hystericis, in verecundia & instante menstruatione, nec non in lactentibus, ab ira nutricis.

8. **Erythema febrile**. Erythema nasi nigricans & pustulosum in febribus malignis mortis instantis signum est. Vide *Necrosis*. Erythema circa nares in febribus non malignis diarrhaeam praesagit.

9. **Erythema ab intertrigine**. V. *intertrigo*.

10. **Erythema complicatum cum alio morbo**. Est rubor, qui tumoribus scirrhosis, oedematosis, vulneribus, ulceribus antiquis, fracturisque supervenit.

Curatur aqua vegetominerali. Erythema ab incipiente *spina ventosa* subinde unguento neapolitano discutitur.

[1] Cel. Theden *Bemerkungen*. 2. *Theil*. p. 253.

Morbilli

Sunt exanthema febrile, quod maculas parum elevatas, rubras, uniformes, in tenuissimam furfurationem abeuntes, format, atque symptomatum catarrhosorum praeludium habet.

Erumpentes morbilli stigmata rubra, elevata, pulicum morsus aemulantia, exhibent.

5. **Erythema ab ictu insecti** [erythema from bug bite]. The most favorable remedy is the application of cold water or parsley macerated in water.

6. **Erythema ab applicatis acribus** [erythema from having applied irritating substance] such as blistering agent, mustard plaster, or caterpillar.

It is treated with unsalted butter.

7. **Erythema volaticum genarum** [transient erythema of the cheeks, flushing]. It is a sudden redness of the cheeks and face, which quickly disappears again. It is observed in those troubled with worms, hysteria, embarrassment, and imminent menstruation, and even in suckling infants, from the wet nurse's anger.

8. **Erythema febrile** [febrile erythema]. Blackish and pustular erythema of the nose in malignant fevers is a sign of imminent death. See *Necrosis.* Erythema around the nose in nonmalignant fevers presages diarrhea.

9. **Erythema ab intertrigine** [intertriginous erythema, intertrigo]. See *intertrigo.*

10. **Erythema complicatum cum alio morbo** [erythema complicating another disease]. This is redness that comes upon hardened tumors, edema related to dropsy, wounds, old sores, and fractures.

It is treated with vegetomineral water. Erythema from incipient spina ventosa is occasionally dispelled with Neapolitan ointment.

[1]Johann Christian Anton Theden. *New Remarks and Experience of Wound Medicine and Medicinal Science.* Erster-Dritter Theil. p. 253.

Morbilli [measles]

Morbilli are febrile exanthems which form slightly elevated, red, uniform spots that resolve with a very delicate scale, and which also have a prodrome of catarrh-like symptoms.

A case of erupting measles exhibits elevated red spots emulating flea bites.

De miasmate morbilloso & de curatione morbillorum vide *Authores* qui *febrem morbillosam* describunt.

Scarlatinae

Sunt exanthema febrile, quod maculas multo latiores quam morbilli, ruberrimas, irregularis formae, prurientes, in desquammationem abeuntes, sine praeludio catarrhali format.

V. *Authores*, qui de *febre scarlatina* scripserunt.

Urticariae

Sunt exanthema febrile quod cum levissima febre erumpit atque maculas parum elevatas, rubras, valde prurientes, & ardentes, cum minimis punctis elevatis, qualia a foliis urticae excitari solent, format.

Illud singulare habent maculae *urticatae*, quod in frigido magis emergant, & in calido evanescant. De *curatione* vide Authores, qui *febrem urticatam* describunt.

Maculae Venereae

Sunt maculae, quae a *viru venereo* proveniunt.

Sunt maculae durae, circulares, rubrae, parum elevatae cum margine calloso, albido, quae in lue confirmata in fronte, circa tempora & in thorace efflorescunt.

Circa frontem formant sic dictam *coronam veneream.*

Curantur interno usu mercurialium & antivenereorum. *Externe* aqua phagaedenica aut solutione sublimati lavari debent.

Esserae

Sunt macula coloris rubri, sed latae, discretae, splendentes, glabrae, ardentes, ac prurientes, planae, *non elevatae* ut maculae urticatae, in manibus & facie utplurimum *sine febre* erumpentes.

For the morbillous miasma and the treatment of measles, see the authors who describe the *morbillous fever.*

Scarlatinae [scarlet fever]

Scarlatinae are febrile exanthems, with spots that are by far more widespread than measles, very red, irregularly shaped, itching, resolving with peeling skin, and it forms without a prelude of catarrh.

See the authors who wrote about *scarlet fever.*

Urticariae [hives]

Urticariae are febrile exanthems that erupt with a very mild fever, forming slightly elevated, red, fiercely itchy, and burning spots, with very small elevated tips, such as are usually produced by the leaves of the stinging nettle.

Urticarial spots have that unique feature that they emerge more in the cold and fade in the heat. For treatment, see the authors who describe *urticarial fever.*

Maculae Venereae [venereal spots]

Maculae venereae are spots that come forth from the *venereal virus.*

The spots are firm, circular, red, slightly elevated with a whitish, callused border, which blossom in confirmed syphilis on the forehead, around the temples, and on the chest.

They form around the forehead the so-called *venereal crown.*

They are treated internally by the use of mercury and antivenereals. Externally, they should be washed with phagedenic water or a solution of sublimated mercury.

Esserae

Esserae are red-colored spots, but broad, distinct, shiny bright, smooth, burning, and also itching, flat, *not elevated*, as in maculae urticatae, erupting on the hands and face for the most part *without fever.*

Subinde in calore laetissime efflorescunt, & in frigore se subducunt, subinde, quod mirum est, recte contrarium obvenit.

Curatio exigit lenia purgantia, dein diaphoretica & diluentia dentur.

Psydraciae

Sunt maculae rubrae in latam ac superficialem vesicam quasi elevatae. Species sunt:

1. **Psydracia spontaneae**, quae etiam *Porcellana* dicuntur, sunt maculae coloris rosei, solitariae, pollicaris diametri, in pectore & brachiis, aliisve partibus tectis subito erumpentes & recedentes.

Curatio exigit purgans antiphlogisticum. Evanescunt sine suppuratione aut desquammatione sola resolutione.

2. **Psydracia urticata**. Urtica urens, cactus, phaseolus pruriginosus & aliae plantae, hanc psydraciam excitant, si manu tangantur.

Cespites vivi applicati cito curant.

3. **Psydracia a punctura insectorum**, a vespa, culice & aliis insectis tales psydraciae oriuntur, quae aquae frigida applicatione optime curantur. V. *Ictus ab insecto.*

Rubedo Cutis

Est rubedo non maculosa sed diffusa per totum corpus vel faciem totam, aliamve partem.

1. **Rubedo a verecundia**. Vasa cutanea genarum a pudore dilatantur, ut in inflammatione.

2. **Rubedo a gelu**. A frigore facies manusque ruberrimae evadunt, sunt qui hanc rubedinem saepe per totum tempus vernale non amittunt. Curatur unguento ad perniones.

Occasionally they blossom most abundantly in the heat and withdraw themselves in the cold; from time to time, which is surprising, the opposite actually occurs.

Treatment requires mild purgings, then diaphoretics and diluents should be given.

Psydraciae [vesiculobullous eruption]

Psydracia are red macules as if elevated into a wide and superficial vesicle. The species are:

1. **Psydracia spontanea** [spontaneous vesicles], which are also called *Porcelain*, are rose-colored, solitary spots, the diameter of a thumb, on the chest and arms or suddenly erupting from other covered parts.

The treatment requires a purging antiphlogisticum. They fade without suppuration or desquamation, by resolution alone.

2. **Psydracia urticata** [urticarial vesicles]. The stinging nettle, cactus, the itch-causing bean, and other plants trigger this psydracia if they are touched with a hand.

Living sod (grass) applied quickly treats it.

3. **Psydracia a punctura insectorum** [vesicles from a bug bite]. Psydraciae such as these arise from a wasp, flea, and other insects, which are best treated with the application of cold water. See *Insect bites*.

Rubedo Cutis [red skin]

Rubedo cutis is redness not in spots but diffuse over the entire body or entire face, or another entire part of the body.

1. **Rubedo a verecundia** [redness from embarrassment]. The cutaneous vessels of the cheeks are dilated from shame (or a sense of modesty), as in inflammation.

2. **Rubedo a gelu** [redness from the cold]. From the cold, the face and hands become very red; there are those who do not lose this redness often throughout the entire springtime. It is treated with the ointment for pernio (chilblains).

3. **Rubedo a vernice**. Sinenses, qui vernicem ex arbore *Rhus* extrahunt, intra 24 horas universali rubore inficiuntur.

Curatur hic morbus ut universalis inflammatio.

4. **Rubedo a venenis**. Esus baccarum atropae & squali caniculae intensam rubedinem per totum corpus diffusam excitat.

Curatur emetico, dein oxymel vel acetum detur.

5. **Rubedo a plethora**. Si homines plethorici exercitio vel calore vel spirituosis nimium se commovent, in facie & toto fere corpore rubent.

Curantur venaesectione, & antiphlogisticis.

6. **Rubedo nativa**. In India incolae insularum Philippinarum sunt atrorubri, & Patagones colorem cupri nativum habent. Etiam in nostris regionibus neunati infantes saturate rubent, at paulatim expallescunt.

Zona seu Zoster

Sunt vesiculae pisiformes, discretae, atrorubrae, non raro confluentes, intense prurientes & dolorificae, quae instar *zonae* seu *cinguli* ad manus latitudinem pectus vel aliam partem circumdant.[1] Cutis simul late rubet, vesiculae serum purulentum continent & apices vesicularum cito gangraenescunt. Sub umbilico & in regione ischiadica usque ad genua hunc morbum vidi.

Peculiaris acrimonia biliosa subesse videtur. Post magnam iram & large desuper potatam cerevisiam his hunc morbum vidi.

Curatur interne dato sale amaro, & externis fomentis siccis. Pinguia & humida, ut vidi, admodum nocent.

Zona herpetica est herpes, quae cinguli adinstar genua aut collum circumdat. V. *Herpes*.

3. **Rubedo a vernice** [redness from vernix]. The Chinese, who extract the resin from the Rhus tree, become infected with general redness within 24 hours.

It is treated as universal inflammation is treated.

4. **Rubedo a venenis** [redness from poison]. The ingestion of belladonna berries or dogfish stimulates intense, diffuse redness all over the body.

It is cured with an emetic; then oxymel or vinegar should be given.

5. **Rubedo a plethora** [redness from plethora]. If plethoric men become affected by excessive exercise or heat or alcoholic beverages, they redden in the face and over the whole body.

They are treated with bloodletting and anti-inflammatories.

6. **Rubedo nativa** [native redness]. In India, the inhabitants of the Philippine Islands are dark red, and the Patagones have a native color of copper. Even in our region, newborn infants are fully reddened but gradually turn pale.

Zona or Zoster [shingles]

Zona are pea-shaped, discrete, dark red, occasionally confluent, intensely itchy and painful vesicles, which, like a belt or sash having the width of a hand, surround the chest or some other part of the body.[1] At the same time, the skin extensively reddens, vesicles fill with purulent serum, and the tips of the vesicles quickly become gangrenous. I have seen this disease below the navel and in the hip region all the way down to the knees.

A particular bilious irritation seems to underlie zona. I have seen this disease in those people who had become very angry and had drunk an excessive amount of beer.

It is treated internally by giving bitter salt and externally with dry, warm poultices. Greasy and moisturizing agents, as I have seen, are particularly harmful.

Zona herpetica is herpes that encircles the knees or neck just like a belt. See *herpes*.

[1]Aliis hic morbus *zoster*, vel *ignis sancti Antonii* vel *erysipelas pustulosum* vocatur.

Macula Lata Plateri

Est macula rubra e pluribus maculis confluentibus constans, cuius ardor tantum est, ut aegri vivam flammam corpus lambere credant.[1] Fere semper pustulis in suppurationem abeuntibus stipatur, & fere nunquam sine praegressa febre calida.

Loca, quae ignis sacer maxime infestat, sunt potissimum alterutrum latus abdominis vel thoracis rarius in facie vel collo vel alia parte observatur.

Ab erysipelate vulgari & bullosa differt suo ingenti ardore, & pustulis suppurantibus, non ut in bulloso, effuso sero exsiccantibus vel in crustas abeuntibus.

Morbus hicce quandoque epidemicus fuit.

Curatio exigit purgantia; ac dein sudorifera antibiliosa vel antiseptica pro ut indoles febris comitis est.

Externe fomentum siccum applicetur.

[1] *Ignis Sacer*, *Ignis Sancti Antonii*, *Hieropyr* ideo etiam ab aliis authoribus haec erysipelatis peculiaris species dicitur. Vide D. Sperlich *dissert. de igne sacro*, *Budae* 1780.

Ecchymoma

Est macula livida, plana vel tumida, successu temporis flavescens, & evanescens, a contusione nata.

Species sunt:

1. **Ecchymoma violentum**, quod ex praegressa contusione, oritur.

Curatur venaesectione & oxycrato spirituoso, aqua Thediana aut fomento resolvente.

[1]This disease is called by others *zoster* or *St. Anthony's fire* or *erysipelas pustulosa.*

Macula Lata Plateri [broad spots of Plater]

Macula lata Plateri is a red spot consisting of several confluent macules, the heat of which is so great that the sick believe that a living flame is licking the body.[1] It is almost always surrounded by pustules that are resolving, and almost never without a preceding hot fever.

The *places* which ignis sacer attacks most commonly are one or the other side of the abdomen or thorax; it is less frequently observed on the face or neck or other parts of the body.

It differs from the common and bullous erysipelas with its intense heat and suppurating pustules, not as in bullous erysipelas, in which effused serum dries up or turns into crusts.

This disease was sometimes epidemic.

Treatment requires purging, and then sudorifics, antibilious medications, or antiseptics according to the nature of the accompanying fever.

Externally a drying poultice should be applied.

[1]This particular species of erysipelas for this reason is also called *ignis sacer, St. Anthony's fire,* or *hieropyr.* See Antonius Sperlich. *Dissertation on Sacred Fire.* Buda, 1780.

Ecchymoma [ecchymosis/bruise]

Ecchymoma is a dark spot, flat or swollen, that turns yellow over time and fades, as a result of contusion.

The species are:

1. **Ecchymoma violentum** [violent bruising], which arises from a preceding contusion.

It is treated with venesection and oxycrate spirits, Thedian water, or softening poultice.

2. **Ecchymoma a venaesectione**. Altero vel tertio die post venaesectionem saepe tota interna antibrachii superficies latissima macula livida suffusa invenitur.

Curatur ut prior species.

3. **Ecchymoma a decubitu**, quod in cadaveribus & in aegrotis diu decumbentibus in dorso & clunibus saepe observatur.

4. **Ecchymoma spontaneum**, quod sine contusione aut scorbuto nascitur. Feminis quibus catamenia suppressa sunt, saepe supervenit.

Curatio est in omnibus ut in ecchymomate violento.

Livor Cutis

Est livor non maculosus sed totam partem occupans.

1. **Livor a strangulatione**. Facies nigro livore sugillatur in supensis fune, in suffocatis, & in neunatis, quibus collum funiculo umbiliculi contortum fuit.

Curatur ut ecchymoma violentum; in infantibus e funiculo umbilicali emittatur sanguis.

2. **Livor febrilis**. In paroxysmo frigoris febrilis & etiam a frigore aeris tempore hyemali digiti & ungues livent. Hicce autem livor sua sponte evanescit.

Vibices

Sunt striae longae, lividae vel coccineae, quales a flagellis relinquuntur.

Species vibicum sunt:

1. **Vibex a flagello**, curatur ut ecchymoma violentum.

2. **Ecchymoma a venesectione** [bruising after phlebotomy]. On the second or third day after venesection, a very widely diffused livid spot is often found on the entire medial surface of the forearm.

It is treated the same as ecchymoma violentum.

3. **Ecchymoma a decubitu** [bruising from bedsore], which is often observed in cadavers and the infirm who lie down for a long time on the back and buttocks.

4. **Ecchymoma spontaneum** [spontaneous bruising], which arises without contusion or scurvy. It often comes upon women in whom the menses are suppressed.

The treatment is in all ways the same as in ecchymoma violento.

Livor Cutis

Livor cutis is livor that is not spotted but takes over an entire part.

1. **Livor a strangulatione** [bruising from strangulation]. The face is marked with a black bruise in those strangled by a suspended rope, in the suffocated, and in the newborn whose neck is entangled by the umbilical cord.

It is treated as in violent ecchymoma; in infants, blood is released from the umbilical cord.

2. **Livor febrilis** [febrile bruising]. In the fit of a cold fever and even from cold air in the wintertime, the fingers and nails will turn black and blue. In these cases, however, the livor disappears spontaneously.

Vibices

Vibices are long streaks, livid or scarlet, as if left behind by whips.

The species of vibices are:

1. **Vibex a flagello** [vibex from a whip]. It is treated as in ecchymoma violentum.

2. **Vibex scorbutica**, vide *maculas scorbuticas.*

3. **Vibex febrilis**, in febribus putridis observantur tales striae, *curantur* ut petechiae.

4. **Vibex a panaritio**. Bis vidi striam rubram a digito inflammato in antibrachium usque pergentem, quae inciso tumore evanuit.

Maculae Scorbuticae

Sunt maculae lividae, quae a scorbuto proveniunt.

In cruribus scorbuticorum non solum maculae *palmares* lividae aut rubentes, sed etiam parvae ut petechiae, & *longae* ut vibices observantur.

Noscuntur ex reliquis signis scorbuti & curantur antiscorbuticis.

Maculae Gangraenosae

Sunt maculae, quae a *gangraena incipiente* oriuntur.

Hae maculae sunt lividae vel nigre, insensiles, in gangraena *humida* molles, in gangraena *sicca* durae sunt. In febribus malignis & putridis saepe tales maculae cum lethali omine observantur.

Curatio exigit antiseptica. Vide *Doctrinam de gangraena.*

Petechiae

Sunt exanthema febrile, quod maculas, pulicum morsibus magnitudine & colore similes, format.

Differunt a veris pulicum morsibus, quod careant stigmate aculei, a pulice infixi, & quod diutius durent: pulicum enim morsus ultra 24 horas non persistunt.

Petechiae febriles a *scorbuticis petechiis* differunt, quod priores febrem putridam comitem habeant. Sic etiam

2. **Vibex scorbutica** [vibex of scurvy], see *maculas scorbuticas.*

3. **Vibex febrilis** [febrile vibex], such striae are observed in putrid fevers, treated as petechiae.

4. **Vibex a panaritio** [vibex from whitlow]. Twice I saw a red streak from an inflamed finger proceeding all the way up the forearm, which disappeared when the swelling was incised.

Maculae Scorbuticae [scurvy spots]

Maculae scorbuticae are livid spots that come from scurvy.

On the legs of scorbutics are observed not only livid or red palm-sized spots but also spots as small as petechiae and as *long* as vibices.

They are distinguished from the rest of the signs of scurvy and are treated with antiscorbutics.

Maculae Gangraenosae [gangrenous spots]

Maculae gangraenosae are spots that arise at the *beginning of gangrene.*

These blemishes are livid or black, insensate, soft in the *wet* gangrene, and hard in the *dry* gangrene. In malignant and putrid fevers, such spots are often observed as a deadly omen.

The treatment requires antiseptics. See the *Teachings on Gangrene.*

Petechiae

Petechiae are an exanthem of fever, which forms spots, similar in size and color to the bite of fleas.

They differ from true flea bites because they lack the mark of a sting inflicted by a flea, and they last for a longer time, for flea bites do not persist beyond 24 hours.

Febrile petechiae differ from *scorbutic petechiae,* because the former may have a concomitant putrid fever.

Color petechiarum est varius. *Rubrae* petechiae boni moris plerumque esse solent, *purpureae, lividae* & *nigrae* pejoris ominis sunt. Rarissimae observantur petechiae ultra cutis libellam *prostantes.*

Ex transsudatione sanguinis putridi ex cute sub epidermidem fieri videntur.

De *curatione* petechiarum vide authores, qui de *febre petechiali* tractant.

Melas

Est morbus, in quo maculae nigrae, vel fuscae, cutem deprimentes, sine dolore & pruritu observantur

Subinde profunde ad ossa usque serpit nigredo.[1]

Est morbus Arabiae endemius, hinc *peculiare miasma* causam proximam huius morbi constituere videtur.

Curatur, praemissis purgantibus, antiscorbuticis, sero lactis cum epithymo vel fumaria & veronica, jure viperino, cicuta, antimonio, mercurio, spiritu cochleariae. *Externe,* synapismi, vesicatoria, balnea sulphurea vel salina, helleborus albus, adhiberi debent.

[1] Vocatur hic morbus etiam *vitiligo nigra* vel *morphaea nigra* seu *lepra maculosa nigra.*

Melasma

Est macula livido-atra, quae tibias potissimum senum absque evidenti causa, & absque scorbuto infestat.

Est morbus diuturnus, qui saepe in ulcera mali moris degenerat, hinc a nomate differt.

Curatio exigit antiseptica interna & externa.

Noma

Est macula rubra vel livescens, quae infantibus vel in gena vel in vulva apud puellas oritur, & intra aliquot dies in sphacelum abit.

Furthermore, the color of petechiae varies. *Red* petechiae are usually the indication of a good prognosis for the most part; *purple*, *livid*, or *black* spots are a worse omen. Very rarely are petechiae observed *standing out* beyond the level of the skin.

They seem to be made under the epidermis from the transudation of putrid blood out of the skin.

For the treatment of petechiae, see the authors who discuss *petechial fever.*

Melas

Melas is a disease in which black or brown spots are observed depressing the skin without pain and itching.

Thereupon, the blackness gradually creeps all the way down to the bones.[1]

The disease is endemic to Arabia, thus a *particular miasma* arising from this region seems to constitute the proximate cause of this disease.

It is treated, after purgation, with antiscorbutics, the whey of milk with epithyme or fumaria and veronica, viper broth, hemlock, antimony, mercury, spirits of cochlearia. Mustard cataplasm, blistering agents, sulfurous or salt baths, and white hellebore should be applied externally.

[1]This disease is also called *vitiligo nigra*, *morphaea nigra*, or *lepra maculosa nigra*.

Melasma

Melasma is a livid dark spot, which attacks the legs, especially of the elderly without obvious cause, and without scurvy.

It is a long-lasting disease that often degenerates into an ulcer with an adverse nature; thus, it differs from noma.

It requires internal and external antiseptic treatment.

Noma

Noma is a red or darkening spot that arises in babies or on the cheek or vulva of girls, and within a few days, it turns into sphacelus.

Morbus apud infantes quinquennes, potissimum in orphanotrophiis, observatur. Haec macula, acu pertusa, non dolet, sine febre oritur, ac sine dolore, tumore, & calore in sphacelum buccae vel vulvae abit, qui sua sponte sine ulla sanguinis effusione partes vicinas & ipsa ossa cum ingenti foetore erodit, & intra paucos dies, pulsu, fame atque caeteris functionibus vix mutatis, mortem causat.

Idem malum subinde scorbuticis supervenit, sed incipit cum ulcere albo & exiguo in interna superficie genae. V. *cancer aquaticus.*

Curatio. Nomae exigit, ut spiritus mercur
ialis saturatus mediante plumaceolo maculae gangraenosae applicetur. *Interne* camphora, cortex, spiritus vitrioli & alia antiseptica dentur.

Nigredo Cutis

Est cutis nigredo non maculosa, sed per faciem, vel aliam partem vel totam corporis superficiem diffusa.

Cutis *nigra* redditur, si humor niger deponitur in cellulas epidermidis.[1]

Species sunt:

1. **Nigredo nativa**, quae in aethiopibus nigris observatur a depositione muci nigri malpighiani. Aliquando etiam in europaeis regio pubis & areolae papillarum in mammis nigrescunt.

2. **Nigredo scorbutica**. Vidi in scorbutico milite totum crus sinistrum adeo nigrum, ut aethiopis esse crus credidisses; curabatur aqua vegetominerali cum spiritu vini camphorato saturata.

3. **Nigredo menstrualis**. A suppressis menstruis manus nigras & lividas vidit Cel. Sagar. *Curatur* ut ecchymoma.

4. **Nigredo necrotia**, qua partes, necrosi affectae, conspiciuntur. V. *Necrosis & gangraena.*

The disease is observed in young children under five, especially in orphanages. This spot, when punctured with a needle, does not hurt, arises without fever, and without pain, swelling, and heat, and turns into sphacelus of the cheek or vulva. This occurs spontaneously, without any release of blood, erodes the neighboring parts and the bone themselves with an unnatural stench, and causes death in a few days, with barely a change in pulse, appetite, and other functions.

The same evil occurs from time to time in persons with scurvy, but it begins with a small, white ulcer on the inner surface of the cheek. See *cancer aquaticus*.

The treatment of noma requires that saturated mercurial spirit be applied to the gangrenous spots with plumaciol. Internally, camphor, bark, spirits of vitriol, and other antiseptics are given.

Nigredo Cutis [blackened skin]

Nigredo cutis is black skin not in spots, but spread throughout the face or other parts or diffusely over the entire surface of the body.

The skin turns *black*, if black humor is deposited in the cells of the epidermis.[1]

The species are:

1. **Nigredo nativa** [native blackened skin], which is observed in black Ethiopians from deposition of black mucus in the malpighian layer. Sometimes even in Europeans the pubic region and the areolas of the breasts blacken.

2. **Nigredo scorbutica** [blackened skin of scurvy]. I saw on a scorbutic soldier an entire left leg so black that you might believe it to be the leg of an Ethiopian. It was treated with vegetomineral water saturated with camphorated spirits of wine.

3. **Nigredo menstrualis** [blackened skin of menstruation]. The celebrated Sagar saw black and livid hands from suppressed menstruation. It is treated the same as ecchymoma.

4. **Nigredo necrotia** [necrotic blackened skin], clearly seen in parts affected by necrosis. See *necrosis* and *gangrene*.

5. **Nigredo sordida**. Aliquando in morbis acutis prospicit cutis, ac si sordes nigrescentes exterius ei insiderent & eam leviter quasi conspurcarent, nullo modo autem hae nigrae sordes se ablui patiuntur.

6. **Nigredo ab ictero nigro**. V. apud Authores *icterus niger.*

[1] Hermann *Dissert. de vera natura cuticulae.*

Alphos

Est leprae species, in qua maculae albae cutem deprimentes nascuntur.[1]

Duplex datur alphi species:

1. **Alphus simplex**, in quo pili cutanei colore non mutantur, sed maculae serpunt de parte in partem, & cutem exasperant.

2. **Alphus leuce**, in quo maculae albidiores sunt, profunde cutem penetrant, pili cutanei albi evadunt, & si locus affectus fricetur, non rubet, si pungatur, aqua lactea effluit.

Causam alphi peculiare miasma, quod Arabiae endemium est, constituit.

Curatio. Leuce vix amplius curatur. In alpho tentari debent eadem medicamenta, quae in melas & lepra laudantur.

[1] Dicitur etiam *vitiligo alba*, seu *morphaea alba*, vel *lepra maculosa alba*. V. Cel. Profess. Vogel. *Dissert de vitiligine.*

Albor Cutis

Est albor per faciem vel totum corpus diffusus.

1. **Albor nativus**. In *Africa occidentali*, homines inveniuntur albi. Vocantur *aethiopes albi* seu lactei, oculi iridem habent roseam, impatientes sunt lucis, debiles & teneri homines, ex aethiopibus nigris, & ex indis rubris nascuntur.[1]

5. **Nigredo sordida** [sordid blackened skin]. Sometimes in acute diseases the skin looks as if blackening dirt has fixed itself on the surface of the skin, defiling it slightly, but in no way does this black dirt allow itself to be washed off.

6. **Nigredo ab ictero nigro** [blackened skin from black bile]. See the authors on *black jaundice.*

[1]Franz Seraphicus Hermann. *Dissertation on the true nature of skin.* 1775.

Alphus

Alphus is a species of lepra in which white macules arise, depressing the skin.[1]

Two species of alphus are given:

1. **Alphus simplex** [simple alphus], in which the color of the skin hairs is not changed, but spots spread around from part to part and roughen the skin.

2. **Alphus leuce** [white alphus], in which the macules are whiter, penetrating deeply into the skin, and the skin hairs become white; if an affected area is rubbed, it does not redden, but if it is punctured, milk-white water flows out.

A particular miasma, which is endemic to Arabia, constitutes the cause of alphus.

Treatment. Leuce is in general seldom cured. The same medicines that are recommended for melas and lepra should be tried in alphus.

[1] It is also *vitiligo alba*, or *morphaea alba*, or *lepra maculosa alba.* See Celebrated Professor Vogel. *Dissertation on vitiligo.*

Albor Cutis [white skin]

Albor cutis is a whiteness diffused throughout the face or the entire body.

1. **Albor nativus** [native white skin, albinism]. In *West Africa*, white men are found. They are called *white or milky Ethiopians*, have pink irises, photophobia, are weak and delicate people, born from black Ethiopians and red Indians.[1]

[1] V. Cel. Profess. Blumenbach *de generis humani varietate nativa.* & Illust. Halleri *elementa physiologiae* T. V. p. 24.

Pallor Cutis

Est cutis praesertim in facie pallor.

1. **Pallor pathemicus**. Terror arterias cutaneas constringendo pallorem faciei & totius corporis causat.

2. **Pallor chloroticus**, qui simul & virescens est, a chlorotica seu pituitosa cachexia pendet. V. *Chlorosis* apud Authores.

3. **Pallor a defectu sanguinis**, qui haemorrhagias magnas & omnes copiosas evacuationes humorum sequitur. *Curatur* cardiacis nutrientibus.

4. **Pallor morbosus**, qui omnes morbos non febriles comitatur.

Maculae Maternae

Sunt macula congenitae seu nobiscum natae. Vocantur etiam *Naevi materni.*

Naevi generatim in *maculas* & *excrescentias* dividi possunt.

Causam excitantem credunt esse vehementem matris gravidae vel cupiditatem vel aversationen.[1]

Multae dantur naevorum varietates respectu coloris, figurae & indolis; frequentissimae *species* sunt:

1. **Naevus lenticularis**. Est macula fusca vel nigra, lentis magnitudine: una vel plures tales maculae praeprimis in facie observantur.[2]

2. **Naevus flammeus**, qui latam maculam, striatam, quae vini rubri in faciem quasi effusi colorem habet, refert.[3]

[1]Johann Blumenbach. *On the native varieties of the human species.* Abr. Vandenhoeck, 1776. Albrecht von Haller. *Elements of Physiology*, Book V, p. 24.

Pallor Cutis [pale skin]

Pallor cutis is pallor of the skin, especially on the face.

1. **Pallor pathematicus** [emotional pallor]. Terror causes pallor of the face and entire body by constricting the cutaneous vessels.

2. **Pallor chloroticus** [green sickness, iron deficiency anemia] is a greenness that happens all at once or slowly develops, resulting from chlorosis or phlegmatic tuberculosis. See authors on *chlorosis.*

3. **Pallor a defectu sanguinis** [pallor from blood deficiency], which follows great hemorrhages and all copious evacuations of humors. It is treated with cardiac nutrients.

4. **Pallor morbosus** [pallor of disease], which accompanies all non-febrile diseases.

Maculae Maternae [birthmarks]

Maculae maternae are spots that are congenital or born to us. They are even called *maternal nevi.*

Nevi can generally be divided into *flat spots* and *excrescences.*

They believe that the inciting cause to be vehemence or desire or aversion of the pregnant mother.[1]

Many varieties of nevi are described with respect to color, shape, and features. The most frequent species are:

1. **Nevus lenticularis** [lentil-like birthmark, mole] is a dark or black spot, the size of a lentil; one or more such macules are especially observed on the face.[2]

2. **Nevus flammeus** [flame-like birthmark, port wine stain] refers to a broad, furrowed spot, which has the color on the face as if showered in red wine.[3]

3. **Naevus tuberculosus**, est macula plus, minus elevata, tuberculis parvis, & non raro ubique pilis obsita.[4]

4. **Naevus cavernosus**, Est excrescencia cutanea rubri vel lividi coloris, quae ex tela cellulosa in substantiam cavernosam mutata, constat, & sanginem vel succum gelatinosum in cavernulis suis continet.[5]

5. **Naevus malignus**. Profundas agit radices, & vasa tumida talis naevi tumorem cancrosae indolis repraesentant, atque causticis multum irritatus in verum cancrum exulceratur.

Curatio naevorum. Partes naevo vicinae emplastro adhaesivo, in quo foramen ad naevi magnitudinem exscissum est, defendantur, naevo autem ipsi unguentum, ex anatica portione calcis vivae & saponis veneti confectum, applicetur. Sic intra duodecim horas naevus in escheram mutatur, quae succedente suppuratione tandem secedit. Naevi tuberculosi facilius, quam maculosi sic sanantur.

Naevi autem magni, quae vera *sarcomata* sunt, etiam ut illa vel ligatura, vel exscissione auferri debent.

[1] Obstetricavi illustrem mulierem, cui mus vivus ex arca, quam subito aperiebat, in mammam insiliit, haec prae terrore animo fere delinguebat atque a tertio graviditatis mense cum tota familia vehementer naevum murinum in infante timuit; praedixi nil timendum esse & praeter omnium opinionem, pulchram, omnique naevo carentem enixa est puellam.

[2] In mamma cujusdam puellae maculam nigram, ut aethiopis est color, aurei magnitudinem superantem, vidi.

[3] Dicitur etiam *morphaea flammea*, germanice *Feuermahl.*

[4] Naevis pilosis muris vel erucae nomen imponunt.

[5] Obstetrices & vetulae his naevis nomen dant rei, cujus similitudinem prae se ferre opinantur. Sic infantes referunt natos, qui *cristam*, *ficum*, *morum*, *rubum*

3. **Nevus tuberculosus** [tuberculous nevus, congenital nevus] is a spot more or less elevated, with small tubercles, and not uncommonly covered with hairs all over.[4]

4. **Nevus cavernosus** [cavernous nevus, hemangioma] is a skin growth of a red or livid color, which, having been changed from a cellular membrane into a cavernous substance, remains firm and contains in its small cavities a sanguine or gelatinous juice.[5]

5. **Nevus malignus** [malignant nevus, skin cancer]. It makes deep roots, and the swollen vessels of such nevi display the characteristics of a cancerous tumor, and becoming very irritated from caustics, it is ulcerated into true cancer.

The treatment of nevi. The areas near the nevus should be protected with an adhesive plaster, in which a hole has been cut to the size of the nevus; however, to the nevus itself should be applied an ointment composed of equal portions of quicklime and Venetian soap. Thus within twelve hours the nevus is changed into an eschar, which finally recedes following a suppuration. Thus, tuberculous nevi are more easily cured than macular ones.

But large nevi, which are true sarcomas, should also be removed in that way or either by a ligature or with excision.

[1] I performed the office of midwife for a well-known woman on whom a living mouse jumped from a box that had opened suddenly. The mouse jumped onto her breast, and the woman almost fainted from terror. From the third month of pregnancy she, along with her whole family, very strongly feared that there would be a birthmark in the shape of the mouse on the infant. I had declared that there was nothing to fear, and contrary to the opinion of them all, a beautiful girl was born lacking any birthmark.

[2] On the breast of a certain girl, I saw a black birthmark the color of an Ethiopian surpassing the size of a gold coin.

[3] It is also called *morphea flammea*, in German, *feuermahl*.

[4] They assign the name of mouse or caterpillar to hairy moles.

[5] Midwives and old women give to these moles the name of the thing whose likeness they think is brought before them. Thus, they report newborn infants

idaeum, *farcimen*, & nescio quid secum tulerint. Hi naevi, cum frigore hiemali contrahantur, & calore vernali dilatentur ob humores rarefactione expansos, hinc opinio confirmatur, naevos, qui fructus referunt, tempore florescentiae: ejusdem fructus, etiam florere.

Maculae Artificiales

Sunt maculae, quae cuti pigmento aliquo inuruntur.

Qui morbos fingere volunt, hac arte utuntur. Sic macula *rubra* solutione auri, macula *flava* hepate antimonii, vel spiritu nitri, macula *nigra* lapide infernali, cuti inuri potest, quae per aliquod septimanas manet, nisi solutione alcalina abluatur.

Colores autem *fuco* inductae ablutione aquosa noscuntur.

~~~~~~~~~~

Cutis Variegata

Est cutis maculis varii coloris deturpata.

1. **Cutis variegata nativa**. In tartarorum gente tigridis instar maculati reperiuntur homines.[1]

2. **Cutis variegata morbosa**. Visa est ad semel in uno subjecto facies viridis, latus corporis dextrum nigrum; & sinistrum flavum.

3. **Cutis variegata a sugillitione**, quae cum solvi incipit, pars maculis flavis, & lividis maculata & striata apparet.

[1] Blumenbach *de generis humani varietate nativa*.
~~~~~~~~~~

who have brought with them a likeness of a *crest* (comb), *fig*, *mulberry*, *raspberry*, *sausage*, and I don't know what else. These birthmarks contract with the cold of winter and dilate with the warmth of spring on account of the humors having been expanded by thinning; from this, the opinion is confirmed that the nevi that remind us of fruit also flourish in the blooming season of those fruits.

Maculae Artificiales [artificial spots]

Maculae artificiales are blemishes that are burned onto the skin with some pigment. Those who wish to feign diseases use this technique. Thus, a red spot can be burned onto the skin with a solution of gold, a yellow spot with liver of antimony or spirit of nitre, and a black spot with infernal stone. The spot lasts for several weeks unless it is washed away with an alkaline solution.

The colors, however, induced by external cosmetics, are revealed by washing away with water.

~~~~~~~~~~

Cutis Variegata [variegated skin]

Cutis variegata is skin disfigured by spots of various colors.

1. **Cutis variegata nativa** [native variegated skin]. In the Tartar race, men are found with spots resembling those of the tiger.[1]

2. **Cutis variegata morbosa** [variegated skin of disease]. This has been seen simultaneously in one subject: a green face, with the right side of the body black and the left side yellow.

3. **Cutis variegata a sugillatione** [variegated skin from bruising], which when it begins to resolve, part of the bruise becomes yellow, and part appears spotted and streaked with dark spots.

[1] Johann Blumenbach. *On the native variety of the human species*. Abr. Vandenhoeck, 1776.
~~~~~~~~~~

Cutis Fucata

Cutis nitida, albitudo cum rosea genarum rubedine, & venis circa tempora caerulescentibus, pulchritudinis exhibet apud Europaeos colorem naturalem.

Foeminae vanae, suspectaeve virtutis, quas natura pulchritudinis colore non decoravit, variis pigmentis hunc sibi inducere tentant.

Fucum *album* sibi inducunt magisterio bismuthi, vel mercurio praecipitato albo, cerussa plumbi, aut remediis cosmeticis.[1]

Fucum *rubrum* praebet carminum. Fucum caeruleum, quo venas temporum sibi pingunt, exhibet succus helliotropii.

Fucum *nigrum*, quo sibi capillos & supercilia nigro colore imbuunt, faciunt solutione lapidis infernalis.

Sed omnes hi fuci, praesertim saturnini & mercuriales, sanitati nocent, & cutem longo usu maculatam relinquunt.

[1] Cosmetica vocantur remedia, quae cuti alborem & nitorem sine fuco seu coloratione inducunt. Haec virtus quibusdam medicamentis inesse videtur. Dilutissima solutio aquosa sublimati corrosivi, bilis, aqua cosmetica Hombergi, aqua cosmetica Hartmanni, aqua destlillata radicis ari &c. huc pertinent. Fumum sulphuris pro dealbandis manibus adhibent.

Cutis Unctuosa

Est cutis splendor unctuosus, ac si esset butyro illita.

Causa proxima est pororum glandularium, vel qui ad tunicam adiposam pergunt, laxa amplitudo, quae oleum subcutaneum transsudare finit.

1. **Unctuositas vulgaris**, curator roborantibus internis, & externa applicatione aquae frigidae & liquoris adstringentis.

2. **Unctuositas elephantina**, quae in elephantiasi observatur, est incurabilis, ut elephantiasis.

Cutis Fucata [painted skin]

Shiny white skin with pink redness of the cheeks and bluish veins around the temples represent the natural color of beauty among the Europeans.

Vain women, with suspect virtue, whom nature has not decorated with the color of beauty, attempt to bring this beauty to themselves with these various pigments.

They apply a *white* dye on themselves with magisterio of bismuth, or white precipitated mercury, ceruse lead, or cosmetic remedies. [1]

Carmine provides *red* dye. Heliotrope juice provides a blue dye, with which they paint on themselves the veins of their temples.

They make a *black* paint with the solution of infernal stone (silver nitrate), with which they tinge their hair and eyebrows.

But all these paints, especially saturnines and mercurials, are harmful to health and with prolonged use leave the skin stained.

[1] Remedies that induce a whitening and brightening of the skin without paint or coloration are called cosmetics. This virtue seems to be inherent with certain medications. A very dilute aqueous solution of corrosive sublimate, bile, cosmetic water of Homberg, cosmetic water of Hartmann, distilled water of arum root, among others, belong here. Some apply sulfur smoke in order to whitewash the hands.

Cutis Unctuosa [oily skin]

The skin has an oily sheen as if it were smeared with butter.

The proximate cause is that the pores of the glands, or those pores which go to the adipose layer, expand in size resulting in the excretion of subcutaneous oil.

1. **Unctuositas vulgaris** [common oily skin] is treated with internal strengthening agents, and externally with the application of cold water and liquid astringents.

2. **Unctuositas elephantina** [oily skin of elephantiasis] is observed in elephantiasis and is incurable, as is elephantiasis.

CLASSIS II. PUSTULAE

Sunt tumores exigui, rubri vel flavi, quorum apex in pus vel crustam purulentam abit.

Sedes materiae morbosae vel in glandulis cutaneis, vel in cellulis sub epidermide esse videtur.

Species pustularum sunt:

Pustulae Solitariae

Sunt pustulae exiguae, quae tempore aestivo solitariae hinc inde in facie, vel in pectore juvenibus fervidis & puellis erumpunt. Utplurimum suasponte suppurantur, exsiccantur & evanescunt.

Curatio, si eruptio valida est, exigit purgantia antiphlogistica, venaesectionem, & externe aqua vegetominerali, vel salita, vel petrosellino in frigida aqua macerato, abluatur facies.

~~~~~~~~~~

Scabies

Pustulas format exiguas, admodum prurientes, quae scalpendo ruptae pus effundunt, crustuosae fiunt; & manus potissimum infestant.

Sedes. Incipiunt hae pustulae forma vesicularum rubrarum in digitorum interstitiis, dein manus, genua & cubitos maximam partem afficiunt, inde per totum corpus, sola facie excepta, disperguntur.

Causa proxima scabiei peculiare miasma esse videtur, quod glandulas cutaneas occupare amat.

Contagium scabiosum vel applicatur corpori, vel in eo nascitur. Hinc primaria scabiei divisio est.
~~~~~~~~~~

CLASS II. PUSTULES

Pustules are small lesions that are red or yellow and on the top of which pus or purulent crust develops.

The seat of its morbid material seems to be in either the cutaneous glands or in the tissue under the epidermis.

The species of pustules are:

Pustulae Solitariae [solitary pustules]

Pustulae solitariae are discrete pustules, which in the summertime, break out here and there in a solitary fashion on the face or chest, in ardent young males and females. For the most part, they spontaneously suppurate, dry up, and disappear.

If the eruption is worthy of treatment, it requires antiphlogistic purgatives, venesection, and externally, the face should be washed with vegetomineral or salt water, or parsley soaked in cold water.

~~~~~~~~~~

Scabies

Scabies forms small extremely itchy pustules, which, having been ruptured by scratching, pour out pus, become crusty, and especially infest the hands.

The seat: these pustules start in the form of red vesicles in the web spaces of the fingers, then afflict the hands, knees, and elbows for the most part, and from there are dispersed throughout the entire body, with only the face spared.

The proximate cause of scabies appears to be a particular miasma, which has an affinity for invading the cutaneous glands.

The scabious contagion is either acquired externally by the body or is born within it. The primary division of scabies is founded on the differences of its origin.
~~~~~~~~~~

1. In *acquisitam*, quae contactu vel concubitu scabiosi, aut gestatione chirothecarum, indusiorumve scabiosi contrahitur. Haec in orphanothrophiis, nosocomiis, & castris perpetuo praesto est, nec non capillamentariis, sartoribus & textoribus familiaris observatur. Huc etiam scabies inoculata refertur.

2. In *spontaneam*, quae sua sponte ab immunditie, habitatione humida, victu acri, salso, pingui nascitur. Haec difficilius quam acquisita curatur.

3. In *criticam*, quae sua sponte tum acutis, tum chronicis morbis supervenit, & illos critice solvit. Huc etiam pertinet scabies catamenialis, quae omni mense loco catameniorum erumpit.

Demum ratione indolis sequentes dantur scabiei *species*:

1. **Scabies humida**. Pustulas rubellas, magnas & purulentas format.

Curatur ut inflammatio cutanea, purgantibus, antiphlogisticis.

2. **Scabies sicca**, quae etiam *canina* dicitur, vesiculas minores & rubicundiores, acuminatas, acri sero plenas, refert.

3. **Scabies herpetica**, qua vesiculas, in albos furfures abeuntes, habet. V. *Herpes*.

Curatio scabiei exigit:

1. *Purgantia mercurialia* saepius repetita.

2. *Antiscabriosa specifica*, ut extractum enulae vel fumariae, conservam fumariae, antimonium crudum, flores sulphuris, decoctum bardanae. [1]

   Externe adhibeatur Balneum ex aqua fluviatili, *Lotio* totius corporis cum solutione sublimati & sale ammoniaco, cum sapone, vel spec. emollientibus, cum radice hellebori albi, aut lotio cum enula. *Unguentum* ex sulphure, vel ex praecipitato albo, vel helleboratum, aut quod efficacissimum deprehensum fuit, *unguentum Jafferi ad scabiem*.[2]

1. In the *acquired* form, which is contracted by contact from either lying with a scabious person or wearing gloves or undergarments of a scabious person. This condition is perpetually present in orphanages, hospitals, and camps and is likewise observed in hairdressers, tailors, and household weavers. In addition, it is also referred to as scabies inoculata.

2. In the *spontaneous* type, it arises on its own accord from filth, a humid environment, and harsh, salty, and fatty diet. These cases are more difficult to treat than acquired.

3. The *critical* type spontaneously accompanies both acute and chronic diseases, and diminishes with the resolution of the disease. Here also belongs catamenial scabies, which erupts every month in the setting of menses.

Finally, by considering their characteristics, the following species of scabies are given:

1. **Scabies humida** [wet scabies]. It forms red, large, and purulent pustules.

It is treated the same as cutaneous inflammation, with purgings and antiphlogistics.

2. **Scabies sicca** [dry scabies], which is also called *canine*, refers to smaller and redder, pointed vesicles full of an acrid serum.

3. **Scabies herpetica** [herpetic scabies], which has vesicles resolving as white scales. See *herpes.*

The treatment of scabies requires:

1. *Mercurial purges* repeated rather often.

2. *Specific antiscabrotics*, such as extract of enula or fumaria, conserve of fumaria, raw antimony, flowers of sulfur, decoction of burdock.[1]

   Externally a bath of river water may be used, washing the whole body with a solution of sublimate and ammonia salt, with soap or specific emollients, with the root of white hellebore, or washing with enula. An *ointment* from sulfur, or from white precipitate, or hellebore, or what was found to be the most efficacious: *Jasser's ointment for scabies.*[2]

4. **Scabies putrida**. Incipit cum vesiculis crystallinis, admodum ardentibus & prurientibus, quae sensim inflammantur, atque in ulcera, magnam copiam puris plorantia, abeunt, ac demum magnas crustas virido-cineritias in toto corpore, nec facie excepta, formant. Inter crustas & excoriationes latae maculae lividae & induratae conspiciuntur. Circa vesperas febricula & ingentes capitis dolores cum rigiditate omnium articulationem observantur. Haec scabies febres putridas sequitur, atque militibus in ultimo bello valde infesta fuit.[3]

Curatur haec scabies: 1. *purgantibus* eccoproticis omni octiduo datis. 2. *Balneis* ex aqua, lacte & sapone. 3. *Oleo vitrioli* diluto & interne dato. Guttae aliquot huius olei in decocto chamomillarum dari possunt. 4. Ulcera & crustae scabiosae unguento albo camphorato emolliuntur.

5. **Scabies topica**, quae in manu, vel alia tantum parte erumpit. Eam optime tollit recens herba *boni henerici*, bis de die imposita quae magnetis adinstar omnem acrimoniam scabiosam ex sanguine extrahit.

6. **Scabies venerea**, quae in fronte & aliis locis papulas duras, in apice suppurantes cum maculis venereis format, curatur mercurialibus ut lues venerea. V. *maculae venereae.*

7. **Scabies verminosa**,[4] est scabies, in qua vermiculi seu acari reperiuntur.

8. **Scabies retrogressa** a scabie imprudenter retropulsa, vel frigore, vel adstringentibus repercussa, multi ac saepe admodum refractarii oriuntur morbi, ut pertinax capitis dolor, vertigo, melancholia, mania, epilepsia, insultus apoplectici, paralyses, surditas, amaurosis, catarracta, fistula lachrymalis, & alii oculorum affectus, asthma, palpitatio cordis, anxietas, ventriculi & intestinorum dolores, obstructiones viscerum, hydrops, atrophia, rhachitis, oedemata membrorum, convulsiones, febres anomalae, magna ulcera cacoetha, magni abscessus subaxillares, & aliae aegritudines.

Curatio scabiei retropulsae exigit revocationem materiae scabiosae ad cutem, vel ejusdem eliminationem e corpore. *Revocatio* saepe obtinetur *vesicatorio, emulsione camphorata, vel succo betulae* per mensem quotidie ad libram epoto, *antimonio diaphoretico, sulphure, fuligine, sulphure aurato antimonii, potu diaphoretico, balneis calidis,* & forti *frictione* articulationum.

4. **Scabies putrida** [putrid scabies]. It begins with crystalline vesicles, with a high degree of burning and itching, which gradually become inflamed and also transform into ulcerations, weeping a great abundance of pus; finally, they form large greenish-gray crusts over the whole body, not even sparing the face. Broad livid and hardened spots are observed among the crusts and excoriations. Around evening time, feverishness and unusually severe headaches with stiffness of every joint are observed. This scabies follows putrid fevers and was very detrimental to the soldiers in the last war.[3]

This scabies is treated with: 1. Purgings with mild laxatives given every eight days. 2. *Baths* with water, milk & soap. 3. Diluted *oil of vitriol* given internally. A few drops of this oil can be given in a decoction of chamomile. 4. Ulcers and scabby crusts are softened by white camphorated ointment.

5. **Scabies topica** [localized scabies], which erupts on the hand or is localized to another part. The fresh herb of good-king-henry removes it best, applied twice a day, which like a magnet extracts all scabious acrimony from the blood.

6. **Scabies venerea** [venereal scabies], which forms firm papules on the forehead and other places, with venereal macules suppurating at the tip, is treated with mercurials as venereal disease. See *maculae venerea.*

7. **Scabies verminosa** [verminous scabies] is scabies in which little worms or mites are found.

8. **Scabies retrogressa** [retrograde scabies]. From scabies being imprudently driven inward, either from the cold or from rebounding astringents, many and often countless refractory diseases arise, such as chronic headache, dizziness, depression, mania, epilepsy, attacks of apoplexy, paralysis, deafness, amaurosis, cataracts, lacrimal fistula, and other ocular conditions, asthma, heart palpitations, anxiety, stomach and intestine pains, bowel obstructions, dropsy, atrophy, rickets, edema of the limbs, convulsions, anomalous fevers, great malignant ulcers, large underarm abscesses, and other afflictions.

The *treatment* of scabies retropulsa requires restoring the scabious material back to the skin, or the elimination of the same from the body. *Restoration* is often obtained by *vesicatory*, *camphorated emulsion*, or by drinking up to 12 ounces of *birch juice* every day for a month, diaphoretic *antimony*, *sulfur*, *soot*, *golden sulfur of antimony*, *diaphoretic drink*, *heated baths*, and strong *massage* of the joints.

His non succedentibus fiat *infectio voluntaria*, dum aegrotus communi lecto, vestibus, indusiis & laquearibus ad detergendas manus scabiosi utatur, vel fiat *inoculatio scabiei*, quae ut inoculatio variolarum peragitur; vel *evacuetur* materia morbosa excitato ulcere, quod *scarificatione*, *setaceo*, *fonticulo*, *inustione*, *vesicatorio*, *exutorio* peragitur.

[1] Cel. Jasser sequentem pulverem omni vespere exhibet rx. flor. sulph. antimonii crudi, nitri depurati, rad. iridos florentinae aa gr. vi.

[2] Ex vitrioli albi, florum sulphuris, baccarum lauri partibus anaticis & oleo lini vel olivarum q. 5. ad unguentum fluidum. Mane & vespere nucis avellanae magnitudo palmis manuum infricatur. Dicit celeberrimus author praemissis purgantibus, balneis & pulvere ad scabiem intra 4 septimanas inveteratissimam scabiem sine omni subsequo malo in aliquot centum militibus fuisse sanatam. Vide Cel. Schmucker *vermischte chir. Schriften 3. B.* p. 169.

[3] Hanc scabiei speciem optime descripsit *Celeberrimus* Baldinger, cui in morborum castrensium doctrina multum debemus, V. Viri hujus doctissimi librum *von den Krankheiten einer Armee.*

[4] In scabie vermes fuisse repertos, nemo, qui Linnaeum hujus rei testem esse novit, in dubium vocabit, dicit *Illustr.* Murray in suo egregio opere *de vermibus in lepra obviis.* Sed hi vermiculi causa scabiei esse non videntur, sed solummodo morbus superveniens. Probabile videtur, quod, antequam scabies in cute erumpat corruptela quaedam humorum semper praecedat, quae si ad certum gradum pervenit, acaros in caseo vel farina latentes (nam ejusdem speciei sunt) allicit, ut in cute nidum quaerant, et rosione sua & excretis liquidis malum reddant pejus. Observamus enim muscas naturae instinctu eam modo carnem invadere, quae jam putrescere incipit. Sic vermes, qui in intestinis nidulantur, non alios, quam quibus peculiaris ad eos recipiendos corporis constitutio est, vexant. Vidit *Illustr.* Linnaeus in lupulo, quod, si ille a larvis phalaenae, radices erodentibus, morbidus factus fuerit, alphides accedant, quae liquido suo, quod ejiciunt, lupulum penitus perdunt.

When these things are not successful, let the infection run its course, while the sick person uses a shared bed, clothing, undergarments, and towels to wipe their scabious hands; or let the *inoculation of scabies* take place, in the same way that the inoculation of smallpox is carried out; or let the morbid matter be *evacuated* after the ulcer has been aggravated, which takes place by means of *scarification*, *bristles*, *fonticulus*,[4] *cautery*, *vesicatory*, and *exutorio*.

[1] The celebrated Jasser administers the following powder each evening: sulfur flowers of crude antimony, purified alkalis, root of the Florentine iris. Six grains of each.

[2] From white vitriol, flowers of sulfur, equal parts of bayberries and flaxseed oil; add a quantity of 5 to a liquid ointment. In the morning and evening, an amount the size of a hazelnut should be rubbed into the palms of the hands. A most celebrated author says that very long-standing scabies had been cured in several hundred soldiers within four weeks with initial purgings, baths, and powder for the scabies without subsequent harm. See the Celebrated Schmucker *Various Surgical Writings*, Book 3, p. 169.

[3] The most celebrated Baldinger, to whom we owe much for the instruction of military camp diseases, has best described this species of scabies. See the book of this most learned man *On the Diseases of One Army*.

[4] Knowing Linnaeus was a witness of this fact, no one will call into doubt that worms have been found in scabies, says the illustrious Murray in his distinguished work, *On the worms encountered in leprosy*. But these little worms do not appear to be the cause of the scabies, but merely a consequence of the disease. It seems probable that before scabies erupts on the skin, it is always preceded by a certain corruption of humors. If the scabies reaches a certain stage, it entices mites lurking in cheese or flour (for they are of the same species) to establish a nest in the skin, and with their gnawing and liquid excrement, they might make it worse. For we observe that flies, with the instinct of nature, invade only flesh that is just beginning to rot. On the other hand, the worms that make a nest in the intestines do not plague anyone else, other than those with the constitution of body particularly suited to receiving them. The *illustrious* Linnaeus saw that in hops if it had become diseased with the larva of moths, with the roots eroding, alphids [*sic*] would approach which with their fluid that they discharge would thoroughly destroy the hop.

Variolae

Sunt exanthema febrile, quod pustulas purulentas, contagiosas pro illis, qui eas nondum passi sunt, format.

Species variolarum tum ratione indolis, tum figurae, tum periculi & decursus valde differunt.

Respectu figurae, quam variolae exhibent, habentur:

1. **Discretae**, si postulae singulae toto morbi decursu ab invicem distant.

2. **Corymbosae**, quae congeriem pustularum densissimarum, non autem in unam penitus confluentium formant.

3. **Cohaerentes**, quae phalanges pustularum, confluentium, solummodo hinc inde sistunt.

4. **Confluentes**, in hac specie pustulae quasi omnes in toto corpore tempore suppurationis in unam confluunt.

5. **Cuspidatae**, pustulas acuminatas formant.

6. **Umbilicatae**, quarum pustulae foveolam, seu umbilicum in summitate habent.

7. **Miliares**, quae pustulas pure vel lympha plenas, sed semen milii magnitudine aequantes, vel paulo majores referunt.

8. **Siliquosae**, quae vesiculas inanes ut siliquas sistunt, ob materiem morbosam ex pustula reabsorptam & interiora petentem.

9. **Bullatae**, quando variolae aquosae confluunt, faciunt bullas magnas seu vesicas lympha plenas, magnitudine nucis avellanae, sub in majores.

Respectu materiae in variolis contentae dantur:

Variolae [smallpox]

Variolae are febrile exanthems that form purulent pustules, contagious for those who have not yet suffered them.

The species of smallpox differ greatly both on account of their nature and by their shape, as well as by their danger and by their course.

With respect to the shape that the smallpox exhibit, they are classified in the following categories:

1. **Variolae discretae** [discrete smallpox], if single pustules stand apart from one another during the entire course of the disease.

2. **Variolae corymbosae** [clustering smallpox], which form a mass of clustering pustules, but not entirely coming together as one.

3. **Variolae cohaerentes** [contiguous smallpox], which present as phalanges of pustules coming together from different directions.

4. **Variolae confluentes** [confluent smallpox], in this species all pustules on the entire body seemingly converge into one at the time of suppuration.

5. **Variolae cuspidatae** [sharp-pointed smallpox], form pointed pustules.

6. **Variolae umbilicatae** [umbilicated smallpox], whose pustules have a small depression or umbilicus at the top.

7. **Variolae miliares** [miliary smallpox], which refers to pustules full of pus or lymph, but equal in size to a millet seed or a little larger.

8. **Variolae siliquosae** [pod-like smallpox], which presents with empty pod-like vesicles, with the morbid material having been reabsorbed and seeking the interior.

9. **Variolae bullatae** [bullous smallpox], when the watery vesicles come together, they make large blisters or bladders full of lymph no larger than a hazelnut.

With respect to the material contained in the pox, the following are given:

1. **Variolae purulentae**, quae pus continent.

2. **Variolae lymphaticae seu crystallinae**, quae vesiculas lympha crystallina plenas sistunt, siliquosae, miliares, vel bullatae esse possunt.

3. **Variolae verrucosae** papulas duras, cuspidatas, verrucis similes, & materiem atheromatosam continentes, exhibent.

4. **Variolae sanguineae seu haemateodeae**, pustulas nigras, sanguinem continentes & fundentes, cum fundo nigro gangraenoso sistunt.

5. **Variolae petechiales**, variolae quaecunque, si in interstitiis variolarum, vel in ipsis variolis maculae nigrae apparent, quae materiem in pustulis contentam rubro colore tingunt, sic appellantur.

Respectu periculi & decursus habentur:

1. **Variolae benignae**, quae regulariter decurrunt, nulla mala symptomata habent, & sine periculo sunt, variolae discretae, purulentae, praesertim insitivae utplurimum sic se habent.

2. **Variolae malignae**, sunt, quae irregulariter decurrunt, quae non maculosae sed papulosae erumpunt, mala symptomata & vitae periculum sistunt, ut variolae confluentes, sanguineae, petechiales, siliquosae.

3. **Variolae regulares**, quae consueta sua stadia regulariter observant.

4. **Variolae irregulares**, quae ordinem consuetum decursus non servant.

5. **Variolae praecursores**, aliquando contingit, ut aliquot diebus ante febrem, vel in ipso primo invasionis die, pustula una, vel plures majores in facie, vel collo vel alio loco erumpant, & confestim pus concipiant, ut in duobus meorum infantum vidi. Hae variolae faustum morbi eventum praesagiunt.

1. **Variolae purulentae** [purulent smallpox], which contain pus.

2. **Variolae lymphaticae or crystallinae** [lymphatic or crystalline smallpox], which show vesicles full of crystalline lymph and can be pod-like, miliarial, or bullous.

3. **Variolae verrucosae** [verrucous smallpox] exhibit firm, pointed papules, similar to warts, containing atheromatous material.

4. **Variolae sanguineae, or haemateodeae** [hemorrhagic smallpox], exhibit black pustules with a black gangrenous bottom, containing and oozing blood.

5. **Variolae petechiales** [petechiale smallpox], and variola of other kinds, are so-called if in the spaces between the pox, or in the pox themselves, black spots appear, which tinge with a red color the material contained in the pustules.

With respect to their danger and course, they are classified in the following manner:

1. **Variolae benignae** [benign smallpox], which run regularly, have no severe symptoms and are without danger; discrete, purulent, and especially spurious smallpox for the most part behave this way.

2. **Variolae malignae** [malignant smallpox], run irregularly, erupt not with macules but papules, and exhibit severe symptoms and danger to life, as in confluent, hemorrhagic, petechial, and pod-like variola.

3. **Variolae regulares** [regular smallpox], which regularly adhere to their own accustomed stages.

4. **Variolae irregulares** [irregular smallpox], which does not keep to the typical order of the course.

5. **Variolae praecursores** [prodromal smallpox], sometimes it happens that a few days before the fever, or on the very first day of infection, one pustule, or several larger ones, erupt on the face, or neck, or in another place, and immediately draw up pus, as I have seen in two of my own young children. These variolae predict a favorable outcome of the illness.

6. **Variolae inoculatorum**, quandoque inoculatores, & illi, qui variolas infantum multum palpitant, unam alteramve variolam in manu sibi contrahunt, licet variolas jam sint passi.

7. **Variolae naturales**, quae infectione naturali.

8. **Variolae insitivae**, quae insitione miasmatis variolosi contrahuntur.

9. **Variolae verae**, quae semel homines aggrediuntur, & intra 14 dies non finiuntur.

10. **Variolae spuriae**, quas sub nomine *varicellarum* sequenti capitulo describam.

Variolae verae, benignae, regulares *quatuor stadia*: 1 stadium *contagii*, 2 *Eruptionis*, 3 *Suppurationis*, 4 *Exsiccationis*, sistunt.

1. **Stadium contagii**, quod cephalalgia, lumbagine, nausea, vomituritione, convulsione quandoque & febre noscitur, ab ingressu morbi ad 4 diem circiter durat.

2. **Stadium eruptionis**. Quarto morbi die primum in facie & manibus, posthaec in reliquis membris puncta quaedam rubra, nunc sparsim, nunc conferta, vel utroque modo usque ad 6 diem paullatim erumpunt, & febris atque reliqua symptomata contagii valde minuuntur, vel penitus remittunt. Sed oris faetor peculiaris, totum conclave adimplens, oritur.

3. **Stadium suppurationis**. A sexto die maculae cutis pus paullatim concipiunt, & in pustulas lenticularis magnitudinis sensim elevantur. Ab 8 ad 11 diem pustulae ulterius ad pisi magnitudinem assurgunt, & depressum hactenus verticem dimittunt. Febris rursum aliquantum increscit, facies nonnihil tumet, fauces dolent, oculi inflammantur, & pustulae suum halonem rubrum amittunt.

4. **Stadium exsiccationis.** Jam per reliquos 4 dies pustulae maturae & flavescentes partim siccantur, partim rumpuntur, & in crustas abeunt,

6. **Variolae inoculatorum** [smallpox of the inoculators] occurs whenever inoculators and those who often come into contact with the pox of infants contract one or two pox on their hand; it may happen even if they have already suffered from smallpox.

7. **Variolae naturales** [natural smallpox], which is an infection produced by natural causes.

8. **Variolae insitivae** [implanted smallpox (introduced by inoculation)], which are contracted by the implantation (inoculation) of variolous miasma.

9. **Variolae verae** [true variola], which attacks people only once, and it does not end before 14 days.

10. **Variolae spuriae** [false variola], which I shall describe under the name *varicella* [chickenpox] in the following chapter.

True, benign, and regular variola exhibit four stages: 1. *contagious* stage 2. *eruptive* stage, 3. *suppurative* stage, 4. *desiccating* stage.

1. **Contagious stage**, which is known by headache, back pain, nausea, vomiting, sometimes convulsions and fever, and lasts for approximately four days from the onset of the illness.

2. **Eruptive stage**. On the fourth day of the illness, first on the face and hands, afterward on the other limbs, certain red papules, sometimes sparse, sometimes close together, or both ways, gradually break out up until day 6; and the fever and remaining symptoms of infection greatly diminish or completely resolve. But a particular stench of the mouth arises, filling up the entire bed-chamber.

3. **Suppurative stage**. From the sixth day, the spots on the skin little by little form pus, and are gradually elevated into pustules the size of lentils. From day 8 to 11, the pustules further rise up to the size of a pea and release their hitherto depressed vertex. The fever again increases to some extent, the face swells in some measure, the throat hurts, the eyes are inflamed, and the pustules lose their red halo.

4. **Desiccation stage**. Now over the remaining four days, some of the mature and yellowing pustules dry up, others burst; they resolve

quae vel sponte defluunt, vel ab ipsis aegrotis decerpuntur. Maculae autem subrubrae in locis delapsarum crustarum subinde per medium annum adhuc remanent, in multis cicatrices seu foveolae in cute, praesertim faciei, relinquuntur.

Causa proxima variolarum est peculiare miasma; morbus utplurimum epidemice grassatur, & qui semel eum est expertus, rarissime altera vice illo prehenditur.

Curatio interna variolarum indicatur a febre, quae illas comitatur. Vide Practicos Authores, qui de *febre variolosa* scripserunt.

Externa variolarum remedia sunt haecce:

1. *Semicupium calidum*, ex aqua & lacte egregie difficilem eruptionem promovet.

2. Palpebrarum coalitus impeditur *lacte calido*, quo oculi frequenter per diem & noctem elui debent.

3. Pustulae in cornea *aqua Saturnina* impediuntur.

4. Ardor faucium *gargarismate acido*, ut syrupo ribium, & spiritu nitri dulci facto, lenitur.

5. Pustulae maturae aciculis, vel forsicula aperiuntur ad evitandas erosiones cutis & absorptionem puris. Facta incisione lactis cremor applicetur.

6. *Crustae aridae*, quas variolae confluentes formare solent, lacte calido emolliri, & dein cerato contegi debent.

7. *Maculae*, post variolas residuae, optime tolluntur oleo been, vel, si aliquoties de die ope penicilli liquore, qui ex aquae rosarum unciis octo, & spiritus vini camphorati uncia dimidia constat, illinantur.

8. *Facies* a variolis praeservatur pediluviis lacteis, atque sinapismis, quae remedia a die invasionis ad initium suppurationis usque adhiberi debent.

as crusts, which either spontaneously fall off or are picked off by the patients themselves. Reddish spots, however, still remain in the places of the fallen crusts occasionally for half a year; in many cases, scars or small depressions are left behind on the skin, especially of the face.

The immediate cause of variola is a particular miasma; the disease for the most part attacks as an epidemic; and he or she who has experienced it once is very rarely subjected to it another time.

The internal treatment of smallpox is classified by the fever that accompanies it. See the practical authors who have written about the smallpox fever.

The external remedies for variola are thus:

1. A *hot half-bath* of water and milk remarkably advances a stubborn eruption.

2. The coalescence of the eyelids is prevented by *warm milk* with which the eyes should be washed frequently throughout the day and night.

3. Pustules in the cornea are prevented by *Saturnine water.*

4. The heat of the throat is soothed with an *acid gargle*, such as a syrup made with currants and sweetened spirit of soda.

5. Mature pustules are opened with hairpins or small scissors in order to avoid erosions of the skin and absorption of pus. After making an incision, cream of milk should be applied.

6. *Dry crusts*, which confluent pox usually form, should be softened by warm milk, and then they should be covered with cerate.

7. *Spots* left after smallpox are best removed with behen nut oil, or a solution which consists of eight ounces of water of roses and a half ounce of spirit of camphorated wine, if they are smeared several times a day with the help of a painter's brush.

8. The *face* is protected from the pox with footbaths of milk and by mustard poultices, which are remedies that should be continuously applied from day one of the infection to the beginning of suppuration.

Fonticuli, vesicatoria nuchae applicata, fomentationes faciei ex aqua calida vel frigida, aut jure carnis vervecinae, itemque inunctio ejusdem cum lardo, vel oleo lini, nec non spirituum applicatio, aut rasura capillorum, & hirudinum applicatio merito ab *Illustr.* & *Expertissimo Professore* Vogel damnantur.

9. Neque mercurius vivus aut moschus in amuleto corpori applicatus speratum edidit effectum.

10. Optima variolas bonas producendi methodus est inoculatio variolarum, sic ex centenis vix unus moritur, aut multum defaedatur.

Varicellae

Seu *variolae spuriae* sunt variolae, quae utplurimum sine notabili febre erumpunt, & intra octiduum iam cursum suum absolvunt.

Differunt a variolis veris, quod febrem vix praecedentem habeant, 2 primo die invasionis erumpant, 3. a variolis veris aegrotos non praeservent, 4. Saepius hominem aggrediantur, 5. Intra octiduum vel citius suum cursum absolvant, variolae enim verae decursus 14 diebus indiget, 6. raro cicatrices relinquant, & tunc maxime pro veris imponunt.

Species varicellarum sunt:

I. **Varicellae lymphaticae**. Sunt pustulae discretae, veris simillimae, iam primo morbi die formantur, humorem continent tenui muco albicanti similem, tertio die siccantur, & ab hoc usque ad septimum decidunt.

2. **Varicellae verrucosae** sive *acuminatae*. Papulas acuminatas, rubras, verrucis simillimas, supra cutem prominentes, in quibus nullus humor est, referunt, & septimo die evanescunt.

3. **Varicellae durae ovales**. Tubercula formant dura, ovalia, obscure rubentia, halone rubro cincta, verisque variolis paulo majora sunt. Post duos vel tres dies nonnihil exulcerantur, & tandem cum nigrore exarescunt, denique pallescunt & subsident. Aliquando sub exsiccatione primo erumpentium iterum novae erumpunt, & sic morbus ad aliquot septimanas protrahi videtur.

The *illustrious and most expert Professor Vogel* properly condemns the following: fonticuli; a vesicatory applied to the nape of the neck; poultices for the face made with warm water, cold water, or meat broth from a castrated male sheep; likewise, anointing of this sort with lard or flax oil; or especially application of spirits or shaving of hair; and the application of leeches.

9. Neither mercurius vivus nor musk applied to the body in an amulet produced the expected effect.

10. The best method for producing a favorable pox is inoculation with variola, thus barely one out of a hundred dies or is much disfigured.

Varicellae [chickenpox]

Varicella, or spurious variola, is a pox that erupts for the most part without a notable fever, and within eight days has already run its course.

It differs from true variola in that: 1. it barely has a preceding fever; 2. it erupts on the first day of the invasion; 3. it does not keep the sick from getting the true smallpox; 4. it may attack a person more often than variola; 5. it should resolve its course within eight days or more quickly, for the true smallpox requires a course of 14 days; 6. it rarely leaves scars, while the true variola leaves scars to a great degree.

The species of varicella are:

1. **Varicellae lymphaticae** [lymphatic chickenpox]. The pustules are discrete, very similar to true variola, already being formed on the first day of the illness, contain a humor similar to a thin whitish mucus, are drying up on the third day, and fall off from this time until day 7.

2. **Varicellae verrucosae** [verrucous chickenpox] or *acuminatae* (acuminate). They refer to pointed, red papules that are very similar to warts, project above the skin, contain no humor, and disappear on the seventh day.

3. **Varicellae durae ovales** [hard oval chickenpox]. They form hard, oval, dark red tubercles, surrounded by a red halo, and are a little larger than the true variola. After two or three days, they become somewhat ulcerated, and at last, they dry up with a black color and finally become pale and subside. Sometimes underneath the drying first eruptions, new ones break out again, and thus the disease appears to be protracted for several weeks.

4. **Varicellae emphysematosae**, quae vacuae sunt ut siliquosae, seu aërem continent.

Variolae spuriae haud raro epidemice grassantur, veris aliquando succedunt, aliquando praecedunt, rarius contingit, ut inter veras erumpant. Periculi fere semper expertes sunt.

Curatio lenia purgantia & diluentia exigit.

~~~~~~~~~~

Terminthus

Pustulae nigricantes & ardentes, quae maxime in cruribus faeminarum observantur, *terminthi* vocantur.[1]

Mox desinunt in crustas, quibus detractis pus emanat.

Terminthi neunatorum. Constant ex pustulis majoribus, quae *lividam aquam* continent, & halonem rubrum habent. Apparent primo ad inguina, inde ad umbilici viciniam, axillas & digitos, & post tres quatuorve dies exsiccatae decidunt.[2]

Subinde epidemice occurrunt, periculo fere carent, nisi maximus eorum sit numerus.

Curatio exigit lenia laxantia. Vesiculae dissecari & dilutissima aqua vulneraria elui, & dein semine lycopodii conspergi possunt.

[1] Nomen habent a ciceribus sive *terminthis*, quos figura & magnitudine referunt.

[2] Ideo germanis vocantur *Schälblasen*
~~~~~~~~~~

4. **Varicellae emphysematosae** [emphysematous chickenpox] have the appearance of empty seedpods or contain air.

Spurious variola not infrequently spreads epidemically, sometimes follows smallpox, and sometimes precedes it, and it rarely happens that they break out with smallpox. They are almost always free from danger.

The treatment requires mild purgings and cleansings.

~~~~~~~~~~

Terminthus

Blackening and burning pustules, which are observed chiefly on the legs of females, are called *terminths*.[1]

They soon form into crusts, from which, when removed, pus issues.

Terminthi neonatorum. They consist of rather large pustules, which contain a *dark liquid* and have a red halo. They appear at first in the groin, then in the vicinity of the navel, the armpits and digits, and after three or four days of drying up, they fall off.[2]

Every now and then, they occur in an epidemic; they are generally without danger, unless the number of them becomes great.

Treatment requires mild laxatives. The vesicles can be dissected and washed out with very dilute aqua vulneraria, and can then be sprinkled with the seed of lycopodium.

[1] They get their name from chickpeas or *terminths*, which refer to their form and size.

[2] For this reason, in German, they are called *Schälblasen*.
~~~~~~~~~~

CLASSIS III. VESICULAE SEU PHLYCTENAE

Sunt tumors exigui, qui pellucidi sunt & non pus ut pustulae, sed aquam, vel serum saniosum continent, atque rupti vel exsiccantur in crustas, vel excoriantur.

Sudamina

Sunt vesiculae granis milii magnitudine & forma similes, subito absque febre erumpentes.[1]

Species sunt:

1. **Sudamina alba**, quae sunt vesiculae concolores cuti, pungentes, & fugaces, quae aestu aeris aut lecti saepe excitantur.

2. **Sudamina rubra**, sunt vesiculae rubrae granis milii magnitudine similes, quae juvenes & calidos viros potissimum tempore aestivo aggrediuntur.

3. **Sudamina balneantium**, sunt vesiculae miliaribus similes, quae in diu balneantibus erumpunt.

Curatio exigit victum refrigerantem. Balneum ex aqua fluviatili, quod eruptionem ab initio promovet. *Lotionem* ex aqua camphorata.

[1] Graecis vocantur *hydroa* vel *boa*.

Miliaria

Sunt exanthema febrile, quod vesiculas granis milii similes format.

Miliaria continent humorem lymphaticum, qui vel excolor est, vel rubellus, pellucidus vel opacus, hinc vocantur miliaria *alba, rubra, pellucida, opaca.* Species miliarium sunt:

CLASS III. VESICLES OR SMALL BLISTERS

Vesicles are small bumps that are translucent and do not contain pus as in pustules, but contain water or blood-tinged serum, and after rupturing, they either dry into crusts or get scratched off.

Sudamina [afebrile miliaria]

Sudamina are vesicles similar in size and shape to millet seeds, erupting suddenly without fevers.[1]

The species are:

1. **Sudamina alba** [white sudamina], which are skin-colored vesicles, prickly and transient, often triggered by heat of the air or the bed.

2. **Sudamina rubra** [red sudamina] are red vesicles similar in size to millet seeds that attack youth and virile men most commonly in the summertime.

3. **Sudamina balneantium** [bath sudamina] are vesicles similar to miliaria, which erupt in baths of long duration.

Treatment requires a cooling diet. A bath of river water promotes the healing of the eruption from its onset. *Lotion* from camphorated water.

[1] They are called *hydroa* or *boa* by the Greeks.

Miliaria [febrile miliaria]

Miliaria are febrile exanthems that form vesicles similar to millet seeds.

Miliaria contain lymphatic fluid, which is either colorless or reddish, translucent or opaque; hence, they are called miliaria *alba*, *rubra*, *pellucida*, *opaca*. The species of miliaria are:

1. **Miliaria febrilia**, quae cum febre erumpunt.

2. **Miliaria lactea**, quae in puerperis, a lacte sano in cutem deposito, oriuntur, sunt alba, & opaca.

3. **Miliaria chronica**, quae sine febre in scorbuto & aliis morbis erumpunt. V. *Sudamina*. De *curatione* miliarium vide authores de febre miliari.[1]

[1] V. Gesner. *Sammlung von Beobachtungen* 3. *Band S.* 104.

~~~~~~~~~~

Hydatis

Est vesicula sphaeroidea, pellucida, indolens, quae pisi magnitudinem habet.

Magnitudine differt a sudamine. Saepius solitaria, quam agminata apparet, in tarsis palpebrarum frequentius observatur.

Species sunt:

1. **Hydatis cuticularis** est epidermidis elevatio in vesiculam aquosam sphaeroidem.

Curatur incisione vesiculae & exsiccatione.

2. **Hydatis cellulosa**, est telae cellulosae degeneratio in vesiculas aquosas, id observatur in quibusdam ulceribus & tumoribus. V. hygroma *hydatitosum* in doctrina tumorum.[1]

[1] Cel. Grashius *tentamen de colica pictonum, cui accedit disquisitio de natura & origine hydatidum.*

~~~~~~~~~~

1. **Miliaria febrilia** [febrile miliaria], which erupt with fever.

2. **Miliaria lactea** [milk miliaria], which during childbirth arise from healthy milk deposited in the skin and are white and opaque.

3. **Miliaria chronica** [chronic miliaria], which erupt without fever in scurvy and other diseases. See *sudamina*. See authors on miliary fever for the treatment of miliaria.[1]

[1] See Johann Augustin Philipp Gesner. *Collection of observations from pharmaceutical science and natural history*. Nördlingen, CG Beck, 1769–1776. Vol. 3, p. 104.

~~~~~~~~~~

Hydatis [fluid-filled cyst, hidrocystoma]

Hydatis is a spherical, translucent, painless vesicle that has the size of a pea.

It differs in size from sudamina, appearing more often solitary than clustered. It is observed fairly frequently on the margin of the eyelids.

The species are:

1. **Hydatis cuticularis** [epidermal hydatid] is an elevation of the epidermis into a spherical watery vesicle.

It is treated by incision of the vesicle followed by desiccation.

2. **Hydatis cellulosa** [cellular hydatid] is the degeneration of cellular tissue into watery vesicles that is observed in certain ulcers and tumors. See hygroma *hydatitosum* in textbooks on tumors.[1]

[1] Celebrated Joannes Grashuis. *Essay on the colic of the Picts, to which is added a discussion of the nature and origin of the hydatids*. Netherlands: Apud Isaacum Tirion, 1752.

~~~~~~~~~~

Vesiculae Crystallina Genitalium

Sunt vesiculae pellucidae, aquosae & dolentes, quae in phymosi & paraphymosi glandi, vel praeputii superficiei internae insident. Hydatidibus sunt similes sed dolentes. Sensim rumpuntur & exanitae corrugantur, aut in ulcera venerea abeunt.

In faeminis autem ex tumidis labiis, nymphis, clitoride ejusque praeputio, & ex vagina prodeunt.

Curantur solutione sublimati vel balsamo mercuriali, si *interne* simul mercurius gummosus adhibeatur.

~~~~~~~~~~

Uritides

Sunt vesiculae latae, rubrae, & admodum prurientes, quae in apice crepant, & ichorem acrem, fundunt.

Utplurimum crura, rarius brachia afficiunt.

Dividuntur in *nocturnas* & *diurnas*.

1. **Uritis nocturna**, quae etiam *epinyctis* vocatur, sistit vesiculas atrorubras, noctu potissime acriter prurientes. Differunt a terminthis, quod ichorem & non pus contineant.

2. **Uritis diurna**, quae *haemeropathos* dicitur, format papulas rubentes, crura obsidentes, quae extra lectum illico apparent & importune pruriunt, in lecto autem evanescunt.

Curatio exigit purgantia & lotiones ex aqua vegetomineralis vel appositionem medullae citri.
~~~~~~~~~~

Vesiculae Cristallinae Genitalium [genital herpes]

Vesiculae cristallinae genitalum are crystalline vesicles that are translucent, watery, and painful, in phimosis and paraphimosis of the glans, or situated on the inner surface of the foreskin. They are similar to the hydatids, but painful. They gradually burst and become wrinkled from having been emptied, or they turn into venereal ulcers.

In women, however, they emerge from swollen labia majora, nymphs, clitoris and its prepuce, and from the vagina.

They are treated with a solution of sublimate or mercury balm if mercurius gummosus is administered by mouth at the same time.

~~~~~~~~~~

Uritides

Uritides are broad, red, and very itchy vesicles, which crack at the tip and pour out an acrid ichor.

For the most part, they affect the legs and more rarely the arms.

They are divided into nocturnal and diurnal types.

1. **Uritis nocturna** [nocturnal uritis], which is also called *epinyctis*, presents with dark red vesicles, itching harshly, especially at night. They differ from terminths because they contain ichor and not pus.

2. **Uritis diurna** [diurnal uritis], which is called *haemeropathos*, forms reddening papules, attacking the legs. These papules immediately appear and itch severely upon getting out of bed, but disappear, however, upon returning to bed.

The treatment requires purgings and washings with aqua vegetomineral or the application of citrus pulp.
~~~~~~~~~~

CLASSIS IV. BULLAE

Sunt magnae & latae elevationes epidermidis a cute, quae vesicas repraesentant magnas.

In hanc classem pertinent.

~~~~~~~~~~

Phyma

Est bulla pure plena, quae utplurimum solitaria hinc inde oritur.

Furunculo est similis, sed planior, mollior & illico suppurans.

Nascitur a depositione puris intra cutem & epidermidem. In pueris & in scabiosis has purulentas bullas frequenter vidi. Nullibi frequentius quam in apicibus digitorum sub nomine *panaritii bullosi* occurrunt.

Curatur incisione, & elutione cum aqua vulneraria diluta.

~~~~~~~~~~

Bulla Solitaria

Est vesica magna, humorem aquosum continens, quae utplurimum solitaria apparet.

Species bullarum sunt:

1. **Bulla vesicatoria**, quae emplastro vesicatorio excitata fuit. Incidenda est, ut aqua glutinosa effluat, sed epidermis non detrahatur. Alias dolentissima sit excoriatio cutis. Emplastro diachilon simplici effluxus seri ad aliquot dies conservari, emplastro albo camphorato excoriatio sanari potest.

CLASS IV. BULLAE

Bullae are large and wide epidermal elevations of the skin, which represent large vesicles.

The following belong in this class.

~~~~~~~~~~

Phyma [abscess]

Phyma is a bulla full of pus, which arises for the most part solitarily here and there.

It is similar to a small *boil*, but flatter, softer, and immediately suppurating.

It is produced from the deposition of pus between the dermis and epidermis. I have frequently seen these purulent bullae in children and in scabious persons. They occur nowhere more frequently than on the tips of the digits under the name of *panaritii bullosi*.

The wounds are treated with incision and washing with diluted aqua vulneraria.

~~~~~~~~~~

Bulla Solitaria [solitary bulla]

Bulla solitaria is a large blister, containing watery humor, which appears for the most part in isolation.

The species of bullae are:

1. **Bulla vesicatoria** [bulla from vesicatory], which had been brought forth by a vesicating plaster. It must be incised so that its viscous fluid water flows out, but the epidermis should not be detached. Otherwise, the removal of the skin might be very painful. The drainage of the serum can be maintained for several days by a simple diachylon plaster; the abrasion can be healed with white camphorated plaster.

2. **Bulla ex ambustione, seu ab affusa aqua fervida**. Incisa vesica applicetur unguentum album.

3. **Bulla a frigore**. Incisa vesica applicetur unguentum ad perniones.

4. **Bullae gangraenosae**, quae in partibus gangraena humida affectis cernuntur, & aqua putrida cadaverosi odoris repletae sunt. Antisepticis ut gangraena curantur.

5. **Bulla pedicularis**. V. *Malis pedicularis.*

6. **Bulla variolosa**. V. *Variolas bullatas.*

7. **Bulla arabum** est bulla sua sponte orta, in diu durantem at exiguam excoriationem cutaneam, cutem sine dolore corrodentem abiens. Folia solani nigri contusa per triduum applicata certissimum sunt remedium.[1]

8. **Bulla dolentissima** est bulla sua sponte excitata, in dolentissimum, at exiguum & diu durans ulcusculum cutaneum abit.[2] Tentetur applicatio contusorum foliorum solani nigri.

[1] Cel. Forskal *desc. plant.* c. 2. p. 46.

[2] Ill. Lorry *tract. de morb. cutan.* p. 424.

~~~~~~~~~~

Pemphygus

Vesicae ichorosae, quae nucis avellanae magnitudinem habent, & utplurimum in variis partibus erumpunt, sic vocantur.

Species sunt:
~~~~~~~~~~

2. **Bulla ex ambustione** [bulla from fire] or from being scalded by boiling water. A white ointment should be applied to the incised blister.

3. **Bulla a frigore** [bulla from the cold]. The ointment for chilblains should be applied to the incised blister.

4. **Bullae gangraenosae** [gangrenous bullae], which are discerned in parts affected by wet gangrene, are filled with putrid water having the odor of a dead body. They are treated with the antiseptics as for gangrene.

5. **Bulla pedicularis** [bulla from lice]. See *Malis pedicularis.*

6. **Bulla variolosa** [bullae from smallpox]. See *Variolas bullatas.*

7. **Bulla arabum** [bulla of the Arabs] is a blister that has arisen spontaneously over a long period of time, but with only light excoriation; the corroding skin resolves without pain. The crushed leaves of the black nightshade applied for three days is the most reliable remedy.[1]

8. **Bulla dolentissum** [painful blister] is a spontaneously arising blister that turns into a very painful but small and long-lasting cutaneous ulcer.[2] The application of crushed black nightshade leaves should be tried.

[1] Celebrated Peter Forskåll. *Egyptian-ArabianFlora. Or descriptions of plants which he discovered and illustrated throughout Lower Egypt and South Arabia.* Copenhagen, Möller for Heineck and Faber, 1775. Chapter 2. p. 46.

[2] Illustrious Anne-Charles Lorry. *Treatise on Diseases of the Skin*, 1777. p. 424.

~~~~~~~~~~

Pemphygus [pemphigus]

Ichorous vesicles are called pemphygus and have the size of a hazelnut, erupting most often in a random distribution.

The species are:
~~~~~~~~~~

1. **Pemphygus febrilis**, qui cum febre putrida erumpit. Vesicae per plures dies manent, tandem rumpuntur & sero ichoroso effuso in maculas atrorubas, crusta nigricante circumdatas, abeunt. Subinde, hae vesicae gangraenescunt.

Curatio exigit primis viis evacuatis antiseptica & acetum bezoardicum.

2. **Pemphygus apyretus**. Hicce morbus in pauperibus sordide & malo victu viventibus sine notabili febre subinde cernitur. Acetum camphoratum prodest.

3. **Pemphygus a tactu colubrid bicephalic**, qui, si vivus vel mortuus tangitur, apud brasilienses excitat vesicas magnas ichorosas, quae tribus mensibus durare solent.

4. **Pemphygus crurum**. Pinguibus, & qui ulcera inveterata in cruribus habent, atque sub sanatione fracturae cruris saepe multae & magnae vesicae aquosae oriuntur in cruribus.

Curatio exigit incisionem vesicarum & elutionem cum aqua vulneraria diluta.

1. **Pemphygus febrilis** [febrile pemphigus], which breaks out with a putrid fever. The blisters remain for several days; they finally burst, and with the ichorous serum having been released, they leave behind dark red spots, surrounded by blackening crusts. Thereafter, these vesicles become gangrenous.

Treatment requires evacuating the alimentary canal with antiseptics and bezoar vinegar.

2. **Pemphygus apyretus** [pemphigus without fever]. This disease is every now and then seen among the poor, living in filth and with a poor diet, without a notable fever. Camphorated vinegar is helpful.

3. **Pemphygus a tactu colubrid bicephalic** [pemphigus from touching a two-headed snake, Brazilian pemphigus], which, if it is touched alive or dead, causes in the Brazilians large ichorous vesicles, which usually last three months.

4. **Pemphygus crurum** [pemphigus of the legs]. Many large watery vesicles often arise on the legs of the obese, on those who have chronic ulcers on the legs, as well as during the healing of a leg fracture.

Treatment requires incision of the vesicles and cleansing them with diluted aqua vulneraria.

CLASSIS V. PAPULAE

Sunt tumores exigui sed duri, qui vel resolvuntur vel ex apice quid humidi ejiciunt, & dein desquammantur.

Differunt a *pustulis*, quod non in suppurationem abeant, a *vesiculis* quod non sint aquosae; sedere videntur in glandulis cutaneis.

Species papularum sunt.

~~~~~~~~~~

Vari seu Jonthi

Sunt tubercula rubra, dura & exigua, quae fere tantum in facie hinc inde oriuntur.

Diu permanere solent, nec dolent, nec pruriunt, nec in suppurationem, ut pustulae faciei solent, abeunt.

Juvenibus victu crasso utentibus, & spermaticis sunt familiares circa adolescentiam evanescere solent.

Curatio exigit purgantia salina & decocta herbacea resolventia.

Externe lotio faciei cum aqua salita conducit. Matrimonium varos curat.

Grutum sive Milium

Est tuberculum faciei albissimum & durissimum, sed admodum exiguum, quod magnitudinem, colorem & duritiem gruti seu milii refert.

Compressione cutis totum tuberculum, quod statim sub epidermide sedem habere videtur, exprimi potest.

Differt grutum ab herpete miliari, quod hic agmen talium papularum referat, grutum autem papulas solitarias.
~~~~~~~~~~

CLASS V. PAPULES

Papules are small but hard bumps, which either resolve on their own or discharge something moist from the top, and then they desquamate.

They differ from *pustules*, since they do not go away with suppuration, and differ from vesicles in that they are not aqueous; they appear to sit in the skin glands.

The species of papules are:

~~~~~~~~~~

Vari or Jonthi [acne]

Vari are red, hard, and small tubercles that ordinarily arise here and there, only on the face.

They usually last a long time; they neither hurt nor itch, nor do they go away with suppuration, as is the case with pustules of the face.

For young men consuming a fatty diet and who are familiar with spermatic function, acne tends to disappear around the onset of manhood.

The treatment requires saline purgings and resolving herbal decoctions.

Externally, it is expedient to wash the face with salted water. Marriage cures pimples.

Grutum or Milium [milium, milia]

Grutum is a very white and extremely firm but very small tumor of the face, which resembles the size, color, and hardness of meal or millet.

By compression of the skin, the entire tumor, which appears to have a seat immediately beneath the epidermis, can be squeezed out.

Grutum differs from *herpes miliaris* because the latter resembles a cluster of such papules, but grutum are solitary papules.
~~~~~~~~~~

Causa videtur esse materia atheromatosa in cutem deposita.[1]

Curatio exigit expressionem gruti ex cute.

[1] Vulgi praejudicium est, grutum cum jure comestum per cutem iterum efflorescere.

~~~~~~~~~~

Herpes seu Serpigo

Est papularum chronicarum ichoroso – squammosarum semper ulterius serpentium agmen.[1]

Species herpetis sunt:

1. **Herpes simplex**, noscitur papulis rubris, pruriginosis, furfuraceis in cute non multum serpentibus, nec eam profunde exedentibus.

2. **Herpes exedens** seu **ferus** seu **esthiomenos**, est herpes qui cutem simul profunde exedit, hinc hic herpes vel simpliciter *ulcerosus*, vel si ulceris labia retorida [retorrida] & dura valde sunt, *cancrosus* est, qualis saepe in facie observatur.

3. **Herpes miliaris**, est agmen papularum, quarum apici rupto inhaeret mollecula subrotunda, flavescens, grano milii similis, unde nomen.

4. **Herpes pustulosus**, est herpes cum pustulis vel vesiculis complicatus.

5. **Herpes syphiliticus**, est herpes, qui a miasmate venereo excitatur, auribus & capilatae capitis parti insidere solet, noscitur symptomatibus venereis, & curatur mercurialibus externis & internis.

6. **Herpes spurius**, qui a causa xterna citra acrimoniam internam oritur ut:
~~~~~~~~~~

The cause appears to be atheromatous material deposited in the skin.[1]

The treatment requires the expression of the grutum from the skin.

[1] There is a belief among the common folk that grutum, when consumed with juice, bursts forth in turn through the skin.

~~~~~~~~~~

Herpes or Serpigo

Herpes is chronic fluid-filled scaly papules that are always spreading further in a serpentine line.[1]

The species of herpes are:

1. **Herpes simplex** [simple herpes] is recognized by its red, itchy, and furfuraceous papules on the skin, neither spreading much nor corroding deeply into the skin.

2. **Herpes exedens** or **ferus** or **esthiomenos** [consuming herpes, or fierce, or devouring] is a herpes that concomitantly eats away deeply at the skin; hence, this herpes is either simply ulcerous or, if the lips of the ulcer are dried up and very hard, it is cancerous, as is often observed on the face.

3. **Herpes miliaris** [miliary herpes] is a group of papules to which, when the tip has been broken off, there adheres a roundish, yellowing little mass of tissue, similar to the millet grain from which it is named.

4. **Herpes pustulosus** [pustular herpes] is herpes complicated by pustules or vesicles.

5. **Herpes syphiliticus** [syphilitic herpes], which is brought forth by a venereal miasma, typically settles on the ears and the hairy part of the head; it is recognized by its association with venereal symptoms, and is treated both externally and internally with mercurials.

6. **Herpes spurius** [false herpes] arises from an external cause rather than an internal acrimony in the form of:
~~~~~~~~~~

α. **Herpes periscelis** est herpes, qui poplitem, ubi zona vinciri solet, infestat, vocatur etiam *zona herpetica,* & a zonae vinctura oriri solet. Curatur zona remota.

β. **Herpes collaris** est herpes, qui collum in forma zonae circumdat. Collum Ecclesiasticorum qui collare acri tinctura vel smalta caerulescente coloratum gerunt, afficit.

γ. **Herpes cerdonum**, qui a sorditie, qua pedes cerdonum perpetuo alluuntur oritur.

δ. **Herpes a tactu Toxicodendri**.

Causa materialis herpetis est peculiaris acrimonia biliosa chronica in glandulas cutaneas deposita.

Causae remotae sunt. Vitium in hepate, ingesta acria praesertim piperata, suppressa evacuatio sanguinis, vel perspirationis, cachexia varia, praesertim scorbutica & venerea, materia febrilis, regio palludosa depressa, labes haereditaria, contagium.

Prognosis. Herpes quandoque criticus est. *Exedens* in cancrum nervosum quandoque abit. *Retropulsus* pessimos quandoque producit morbos: inflammationem pectoris, phthisin, tumorem cancroidem &c.

Curatio requirit purgantia & depurantia sanguinis serum. Mercurius vivus cum sulphure aurato praeprimis se commendat.[2] In herpete exedente acidum vitrioli interne & externe adhibitum, esus pomorum acidorum profuit.[3] Fumaria, sarsaparilla, dulcamara, jus viperae, antimonialia, cicuta, spiritus salis acidus, mercurius gummosus, dulcis, sublimatus, aquae martiales acidulae, cortex peruvianus cum asseclis mixtus.

Externe oleum tartari per deliquium, aut unguentum rosaceum cum sulphure, mercurio praecipitato albo, vel floribus zinci, aut benzoes laudatur. Nec non radix lapati in aceto macerata, thermae sulphureae, aqua marina, aqua vegeto mineralis cum spiritu vitrioli, balneum e scoriis metallorum, solutio ex vitriolo albo, sale communi, sulphure, alumine. Aqua stillatitia e succo pomorum borsdorfensium. Folia boni henrici, oleum palmae. Creta

α. **Herpes periscelis** [herpes of the garter] is herpes, which attacks the thigh or knee, where the belt is usually bound; this herpes is also called *zona herpetica* (belt herpes), and is likely to arise from the binding of a garter. It is cured by removing the garter.

β. **Herpes collaris** [herpes of the collar] is herpes that goes around the neck in the shape of a belt. It is herpes that affects the neck of ecclesiatics, who wear a collar with a stinging dye or deep-blue pigment.

γ. **Herpes cerdonum** [herpes of the craftsman], which arises from filth, which with the feet of craftsmen are constantly in contact.

δ. **Herpes a tactu toxicodendri** [herpes from touching poison ivy]

The material cause of herpes is a particular chronic bilious acrimony deposited in the cutaneous glands.

The remote causes are: a liver defect; having ingested spicy food, especially peppers; suppressed evacuation of the blood or sweat; various wasting diseases—especially scurvy and venereal disease; substances employed for reducing fever; living in low-lying, swampy areas; hereditary defects; and contagion.

Prognosis. Herpes is sometimes critical. Herpes sometimes turns into a vigorous cancer. Driving it inward sometimes produces the worst diseases: inflammation of the chest, phthisis, a cancerous tumor, etc.

The treatment requires purgings and purifying of blood serum. Mercurius vivus with golden sulfur is especially recommended.[2] In herpes exedens, acid of vitriol employed internally and externally and eating acidic fruit is beneficial.[3] Peruvian bark mixed with the following: fumaria, sarsaparilla, climbing nightshade, viper broth, antimonials, hemlock, acidic spirit of salt, gummy sweet mercury sublimate, and slightly sour martial water.

Externally, oil of tartar per deliquium or rose ointment with sulfur, white mercury precipitate, and either flowers of zinc or benzoes are recommended. And also the root of the bitter dock soaked in vinegar, sulfur baths, seawater, vegetomineral water with the spirits of vitriol, a bath of metal dross, a solution of white vitriol with common salt, sulfur, and alum. Water drippings from the juice of the borsdorf apple. The leaves of the good-king-henry, palm oil.

cum lactis cremore, plumbata, mercurialia praesertim solutio sublimati, fonticulus, caustica, lavatorium ex radice hellebori albi & his medicamentis non sufficientibus, emplastrum vesicatorium super parte herpetica applicatum, efficacissima herpetis remedia deprehendi.[4]

[1] D. Pitner *diss. de herpete. Budae*, 1780.

[2] Schmucker *vermischte chirurg. Schriften*, S. 63.B. 1.

[3] *Collectanea Societatis medicae Havniensis* T. II. p. 1

[4] Blochs, *medicinische Bemerkungen* S. 97.

~~~~~~~~~~

Cutis Anserina

Cutis subito & ubique innumeris tuberculis, minimis, pallidis, repletur, qualia in cute anserum observantur.

Causa proxima est contractio textus fibrosi cutanei, quae papillas cutaneas protrudit.

Hinc a frigore ad corpus calefactum admisso, a terrore, a spasmo cutaneo febris intermittentis, & etiam post mortern in cadavere observatur.

Curatio. Est morbus fugax, calore brevi & sua sponte evanescens.

~~~~~~~~~~

Tuberculum

Est tumor induratus, subcutaneus, cuti concolor, papula major, non tamen adeo magnus, ut ad tumores magnos referri potius possit.

Species tuberculorum sunt:

1. **Tuberculum scirrhosum**, quod induratio seu scirrhus glandulae subcutaneae est, sed benignus, indolens, & cuti concolor. Cancer mammarum saepe a parvo tali tuberculo, per multos saepe annos quiete

Chalk with cream of milk with lead, and mercurials, especially a solution of sublimate, fonticulus, caustics, white hellebore root bath. When these treatments are not sufficient, I have found a vesicatory plaster applied on top of the herpetic area to be the most effective remedy for herpes.[4]

[1] Gabriel Pitner. *Dissertation on Herpes.* Budae: Landerer, 1780.

[2] Johann Leberecht Schmucker. *Miscellaneous Surgical Writings.* p. 63. Volume 1.

[3] *Collection of the Medical Society of Copenhagen.* Medicinske Selskab. 1774. Book II, p. 1.

[4] Marcus Bloch. Medical Remarks. p. 97.

~~~~~~~~~~

Cutis Anserina [goosebumps]

Cutis anserina is observed when suddenly and everywhere, the skin is filled with innumerable tiny, pale papules, like the skin of the goose.

The immediate cause is a contraction of the cutaneous fibrous tissue, which protrudes the cutaneous bumps.

It is observed from these causes: when cold comes in contact with a warm body, or when a person experiences terror, or from skin spasm with intermittent fevers, and even after death in cadavers.

Treatment. It is a fleeting disease, disappearing quickly and spontaneously with warmth.

~~~~~~~~~~

Tuberculum [tubercles, nodules]

A tubercle is an indurated, subcutaneous, skin-colored, rather sizeable papule, not so big, however, that it can instead be categorized with the large tumors.

The species of tubercles are:

1. **Tuberculum scirrhosum** [scirrhous nodule], which is an induration or hardness of subcutaneous glands, but is benign, painless, and skin-colored. Cancer of the breast often starts with just such a small tubercle,

haerente, incipit, quod cessantibus menstruis, aut irritatione externa saepe in magnum carcinoma mutatur.

2. **Tuberculum cancrosum**, quod etiam *noli me tangere* vocatur, est parvum tuberculum in facie, rubrolividum, quod per multos annos quietum manet, si vero medicamentis multum irritatur, dolere incipit & in pessimum cancrum nerveum faciei abit.

3. **Tuberculum cisticum**, est parvus tumor subcutaneus, atheromatosus vel sevosus, qui saepe per totam vitam vel manet, vel in atheroma abit.

4. **Tuberculum scrophulosum**. Scrophulae colli cum parvis talibus tuberculis, quae circa venam jugularem externam rosarii adinstar descendunt, incipiunt.

5. **Tuberculum leprosum**. Format lepra tubercula squammosa & crustosa in toto corpore & facie. V. *lepra.*

6. **Tuberculum sarcoticum**. Mollia, rubra & indolentia talia tubercula saepe magno numero in naso propullulant.

7. **Tuberculum hydatitosum**. Hydatides subcutaneae, in scroto vel sub mamma nascentes, globulos rotundos & durissimos referunt.

8. **Tubercula pannoica**, quae ab Hungaris *Tsömör* vocantur; languore, & nausea praegressa oriuntur tubercula, quae tactu manifestantur, circa tempora, in dorso, nucha, brachiis, praesertim in collo & carpo manuum.

Curantur laxantibus, & dein datis diaphoreticis.

Externe convenit frictio tuberculorum cum allio & aceto vini.[1]

Curatio. Tubercula juxta indolem tumoris, quem referunt, curari debent. Vide *Doctrinam de tumoribus.*

[1] Baty *Specimen morborum Hungaris endemiorum.*

often remaining dormant for many years; after menopause or external irritation, it often changes into a large carcinoma.

2. **Tuberculum cancrosum** [cancerous tubercle, skin cancer], also called *noli me tangere* [touch me not], is a small darkish-red nodule on the face. Even though it may remain quiet for many years, if it is irritated too much by medications, it begins to hurt and turns into a most vigorous cancer of the face.

3. **Tuberculum cisticum** [cystic tubercle] is a small subcutaneous atheromatous or sebaceous tumor that often either remains as such throughout a person's entire life or turns into an atheroma.

4. **Tuberculum scrophulosum** [scrofulous tubercle]. Scrofula of the neck begins with such small nodules, which descend around the external jugular vein like a rosary.

5. **Tuberculum leprosum** [leprous tubercle]. Lepra forms scaly and crusty nodules over the entire body and face. See *lepra*.

6. **Tuberculum sarcoticum** [fleshy tubercle]. Soft, red, and painless nodules sprout on the nose often in great numbers.

7. **Tuberculum hydatitosum** [hydatid tubercle]. Refers to round, globular, and very firm subcutaneous hydatids, beginning on the scrotum or under the breasts.

8. **Tubercula pannoica** [Pannonian tubercle], which by the Hungarians are called *Tsömör*, are nodules that arise with weakness and preceding nausea, brought about by picking around the temples, the back, nape of the neck, arms, and especially around the neck and wrists.

They are treated with laxatives and then by giving diaphoretics.

Externally it is appropriate to rub the tubercles with garlic and wine vinegar.[1]

Treatment. Tubercles should be treated according to the nature of the tumor from which they get their name. See the *teachings on tumors*.

[1] Joannes Baty. *Inaugural medical specimen containing a description of certain diseases endemic to Hungary and the remedies for the same, familiar and quasi-domestic.* Netherlands: ex officina Abrahami van Paddenburg, 1775.

Phygethlon

Est tuberculum rubrum & dolens, quod varo majus, furunculo minus, & phymate durius est.

Saepe circa anum tale tuberculum oritur, quod male tractarum in fistulam ani abit.

Curatio exigit purgantia & externe aquam vegetomineralem.

~~~~~~~~~~

Lepra

Est morbus in quo cutis praesertim faciei rugosa, & aspera evadit, atque tuberibus magnis rubro-lividis & rimosis deformatur, cum extremorum artuum insensilitate & voce rauca nasali.[1]

Signa. Incipit morbus cum una rarius pluribus maculis minimis: morbus incipiens ex cutis insensilitate & maculis rubro-pallidis, acus puncturam vix superantibus, quae aegre a lentigine dinstinguuntur, quod tamen ope acus adhibitae, quae infixa nullum dolorem excitat, & animadversione, an increscat, fieri potest, noscitur.

Hae maculae sine omni inflammatione & elevatione sed potuis [sp. probably potius] cum depressione paullatim dilatantur.

Simul cum maculis auricularum lobi intumescunt & indurantur, atque in toto ambitu subinde tuberculis cinguntur. Deinde nares, labia oris & universa facies turgescunt & rubore quodam quasi cinnabarino inficiuntur, progressu temporis ad caeruleum vergente, & in vetustiori morbo lividiore evadente. Cutis praeterea adest insensilis, & in rugas obdurescentes corrugatur.

Excreta sana sunt, urina tamen pallidula, muriam halecum olet, citoque putrescit. Sic morbus quandoque sine notabili incremento per X vel XX annos subsistit. Si vero non bona adhibeatur diaeta, tunc Maculae leprosae a facie per universum corpus ad plantas pedum usque erumpunt, atque in tubera, habitum corporis mirifice deformania, surgunt. Maxime sub unguibus nascuntur vesiculae, apices digitorum crassescunt & sensum amittunt, serpit e prima phalange malum in alteram citra dolorem, atque ossicula absque dolore delabuntur.
~~~~~~~~~~

Phygethlon [abscess]

Phygethlon is a red and painful nodule that is larger than a varus, smaller than a furuncle, and firmer than a phyma.

Such a nodule often arises around the anus, and after being ineptly handled, it turns into an anal fistula.

The treatment requires purging and externally vegetomineral water.

~~~~~~~~~~

Lepra

Lepra is a disease in which the skin, especially of the face, is wrinkled and becomes rough and even deformed by large, reddish-livid and fissured nodules, with the joints of the extremities numb and the voice raspy and nasal.[1]

Signs. The disease begins with one or—more rarely—very many tiny spots. The incipient disease is recognized by insensate skin and reddish-pale spots barely bigger than a prick of a needle, which in the affected person are scarcely distinguished from a freckle. However, the disease is confirmed by means of an inserted needle that causes no pain; it is possible to determine by observation whether the pain increases as it is inserted more deeply.

These macules are without any inflammation and elevation but rather expand little by little and become indented.

At the same time, the lobes of the ears swell and become indurated with macules, and thereupon, the lobe is completely encircled with nodules. Then the nares, the lips, and the whole face begin to swell and become affected with a certain redness as if stained with cinnabar, progressing over time to a bluish color, and turning more livid later in the disease. The skin is henceforth insensate and corrugated with hardening wrinkles. The excretions are healthy; however, the pallid urine smells of briny fish and quickly putrefies. Thus at this stage the disease sometimes remains without notable worsening for 10–20 years.

But if the person is not adhering to a good regimen, then lepromatous macules erupt all the way from the face, throughout the entire body to the soles of the feet; they rise into nodules, remarkably deforming the appearance of the body. Vesicles arise chiefly under the nails, thickening the tips of the digits, and taking away their sensation; the malady creeps from the first phalange to another without pain, going down the bones without pain.
~~~~~~~~~~

Interdum universum corporis integumentum induratur & ob transpirationem penitus suppressam intumescit in leucophlegmatiam. Accedunt ulcera anodyna, quae densis crustis brevi labentibus & renascentibus obteguntur. Haec ulcera interdum, quum cutis in toto maculae ambitu consumpta esset, sine ulla medela consolidantur, dum paullo post aliae maculae prodeunt, quae pariter exulcerantur. Quidquid e corpore humoris transpirat, intolerabiliter foetet. Pertinax adest obstipatio, excrementa sunt nigra, valde sicca. Urina rufa, uroscopiis tenaciter adhaerens. Sitis perpetua: lingua semper sicca, interdum nigris crustis tecta, & hinc inde quasi rimosa. Sanguis admodum tenuis, exiguam seri copiam dimittit, & ex vena missus putridum olet, cruoris globuli sunt albi. Stimulus ad veneream assidu & cum genitalium pruritu ad mortem usque non coërcibilis.

Causa proxima est miasma seu acrimonia sui generis, lentam putredinem humorum & languorem cutis & extremorum inducens. Morbus inter Arabes, Aegyptios, Abyssiniam & Americam meridionalem endemius, & frequens est. Contrahitur a parentibus & per ubera, coitum, habitum, & sudorem subjecti morbosi: etiam domicilia infecta aliis sunt contagiosa.

Causae excitantes esse censentur esus carnium semiputridarum: victus piscium & porcorum pinguium leprosorum: potus aquae multis piscibus putrescentibus repletae: tempestas constans calida, sicca vel in summo gradu humida. Terror, veneris abusus, refrigeratio contagium jam receptum cito & saepe intra unam noctem evoluunt.

Prognosis. Lepra est vera crisis virus leprosi, hinc toleranda. Recens curabilis, adulta incurabilis est.[2]

Curatio exigit, ut causae excitantes & causae morbum adaugentes fugentur.

Crisis per cutim promovenda ope balneorum tepidorum, bis in septimana ad 15 horae minuta usurpatorum, dein quotidie bis adhibitorum, cum emollientibus & leniter detergentibus: ut hepate sulphuris in aqua soluto, exercitatione & vino promotis per trimestre adhibitis.

Ulcera tinctura aloes, myrrhae & succini deligentur. *Calli* cutis unguento de althea & enulae emolliantur.

Sometimes, the entire surface of the skin of the body is hardened and becomes swollen into anasarca from transpiration forced inward. Painless ulcers develop, which are covered over in dense crusts that in a brief time fall off and regenerate. Sometimes these ulcers, when the skin has been consumed in total by a confluence of macules, are consolidated without any remedy, while a little later other macules appear, which likewise ulcerate. Whatever humor transpires from the body, it stinks intolerably. Persistent constipation is present, with the feces black and very dry. The urine is ruddy, adhering tenaciously to the uroscopes. Perpetual thirst: the tongue is always dry, sometimes covered in black crusts, and as a result, it is as if the tongue is full of cracks. The blood is extremely thin, sending an inadequate supply of serum; when released from the vein it smells putrid, and there are white globules in the blood. Constant stimulation of the sex organs and itching of the genitals up until death cannot be controlled.

The proximate cause is a miasma or acrimony of its own kind, inducing a slow putrefaction of the humors and weakness of the skin and extremities. The disease is endemic and frequent among Arabs, Egyptians, Abyssinians, and South Americans. It is contracted from parents and through the lactating breast, through coitus, through clothing, and through sweat of diseased subjects; even the domiciles of the infected are contagious to others.

Promoting causes are considered to be the eating of semiputrid meats; a diet of fatty and leprous fish and pork; the drinking of water replete with many rotting fish; a climate consistently warm, dry, or extremely humid. After having received the contagion, terror, wasting of the genitals, and coolness quickly and often evolve in one night.

Prognosis. Lepra is a true crisis of the leprous virus and hence must be eradicated from the body. The recently infected are curable, but those with the disease at its peak are incurable.[2]

Treatment requires that stimulating causes and those that worsen the disease be eliminated.

A decisive change for the skin must be induced with the help of warm baths, twice a week for 15 minutes of use, then twice daily applications with emollients, gently wiped off: such as liver of sulfur dissolved in water, enhanced by exercise and wine, employed for three months.

The *ulcers* should be bandaged with tincture of aloe, myrrh, and amber. The skin's calluses should be softened with ointment of althea and enula.

Si morbus fugatus, corpus roborandum interne & externe per suffimigia. *Antileprosa* interne danda.

In sanatis maculae distinctae non amplius increscentes a lepra remanent.

Curatio interna tentari potest ledo palustri,[3] aethiope minerali, antimonio, croco martis, lacte, purgantibus.

Externe adhibeantur solutio salis ammoniaci, balnea sulphurea, martialia, helleborata, & inungantur crustae butyro, vel unguento ad lepram.[4]

Lepra asturiensis, est lepra Asturiensibus endemia, in qua crustae aestivo tempore delabuntur & cicatrices coloris rosei, infra cutis libellam depressas, lucidas & per vitam durantes reliquunt. Malum insanabile censetur.

Demum multi alii morbi cutanei, qui pertinaces sunt & totum fere corpus occupant, nomine leprae ab Authoribus denotantur, ut

1. **Lepra herpetica**, est herpes crustaceus in toto corpore. V. *Herpes.*

2. **Lepra scabiosa** est scabies putrida, quae etiam totum corpus occupat. V. *Scabies putrida.*

3. **Lepra fungifera**, quae excrescentias fungosas format. V. *Frambaesia.*

4. **Lepra sqammosa** [*sic*], quae ubique squammas producit. V. *Ichtyosis* [*sic*] & *impetigo.*

5. **Lepra maculosa**, seu vitiligo quae maculis depressis, albis vel nigricantibus cutem defaedat. V. *Alphos* & *Melas.*

6. **Lepra elephantiaca seu arabica**. V. *Elephantiasis.*

7. **Lepra setosa**, vide *hystriciasis.*

8. **Lepra topica**, quae unam solummodo partem afficit.

[1] Cel. Schilling, *de lepra*, Lugd. Batav. 1778.

If the disease is put to flight, the body must be strengthened internally and externally through fumigation. *Antileprotics* should be given internally.

In the cured, the distinct blemishes from lepra remain, no longer increasing.

An internal treatment can be attempted with wild rosemary,[3] Ethiopian minerals, antimony, crocus martis, milk, and purgings.

Externally employed are: ammonium chloride solution, sulfurous baths, martial baths, and helleborate baths, and the crusts should be anointed with butter or ointment for lepra.[4]

Asturian lepra is lepra endemic to the Asturians, in which crusts fall off during the summertime and leave scars of pink color, depressed below the level of the skin, bright and hardening throughout life. It is considered an incurable malady.

Finally, there are many other skin diseases which are obstinate and occupy almost the entire body and are given by authors the name of lepra:

1. **Lepra herpetica** [herpetic lepra] is crustaceous herpes over the entire body. See *Herpes.*

2. **Lepra scabiosa** [scabious lepra] is putrid scabies, which also takes over the entire body. See *Scabies putrida.*

3. **Lepra fungifera** [fungiform lepra], which forms fungous growths. See *Frambaesia.*

4. **Lepra squammosa** [squamous lepra, psoriasis], which produces scales everywhere. See *Ichthyosis* and *impetigo.*

5. **Lepra maculosa** [macular lepra], or vitiligo, which disfigures the skin with depressed white or blackening spots. See *alphos* and *melas.*

6. **Lepra elephantiaca or Arabica** [Arabian lepra]. See *Elephantiasis.*

7. **Lepra setosa** [bristled lepra], see *hystriciasis.*

8. **Lepra topica** [localized lepra], which affects only one part.

[1] G. W. Schilling. *Commentaries on Leprosy.* Leiden, 1778.

[2] Facilius sanatur lepra, quae totum corpus, quam quae solum partem afficit. Acida & mercurialia leprosis noxia sunt.

[3] *Schwedische Abh.* 35. vol. Cel. Odhelins casum refert ancillae lepra nodulosa affectae, in qua ex infuso ledi palustris seu roris marini sylvestris nodi sensim resoluti fuerunt.

[4] Florentiae in nosocomio S. Eusebii leprosi omni altero die inunguntur & sic sine alio fere remedio curantur, sequenti unguento: Rx. Lardi & butyri majalis aa ℔iiʃs Terebinthinae ℥xiv cerae albae ℥ij. liquefiant lento igne; dein adde, mercurii praecipitati rubri ℥j. Salis communis sicci & merc. sublimati corrosivi aa ℥ij. Succi limoniorum & spiritus aceti aa q. s. pro unguento formando. V. Galeoti [sic] *Dissertatione sopra les malattie, che si curano nel regio spedale di S. Eusebio con i rimedi soliti usarsi nel medesimo.* Firenze 1771.

Elephantiasis

Est lepra, quae potissimum pedes afficit.[1]

Signa. In pede adfecto phalanges ossiculorum paullatim intumescunt, cutim & carnes mirum in modum expandunt, crassescunt digiti, tandemque colliquescunt cerae adinstar, unde a levissima causa haemorrhagia, sponte & cito iterum cessans. Serpit malum ad femur usque, contracturam articulorum efficiens.

Simul panniculus adiposus & cutis in plicas & rugas ita sensim se componunt, ut pedis elephantini formam omnino referat. Demum cruribus deformatis & manuum digiti circa articulos tument, & successive soluti cadunt, inde absque dolore ulcera primo faciem & dein carnosas partes cum intolerabili foetore depascuntur.

Anatome in amputato ejusmodi crure nulla periostii externi & medullae ossium vestigia, nec ullas cavitates ossium deprehendit. Nulla ferme vasa vel sanguifera vel lymphatica in partibus internis observantur, eaque in corrugata cute sunt varicosa & fere inania, ambo cruris ossa & ossa pedum quasi in unum confluxerunt, & arteria interossea est deleta.

[2] Lepra which affects the whole body is more easily cured than that which affects only one part. Acids and mercurials are noxious to lepra.

[3] Erik Odhelins. *Transactions of the Royal Swedish Academy of Sciences.* Vol. 35. Reports a case of nodular lepra affecting a maidservant, in which the nodules were resolved slowly from an infusion of rosemary of the swamp or forest.

[4] In Florence at the infirmary of St. Eusebius, lepers are rubbed every other day; thus without almost any other remedy, they are cured with the following ointment: Recipe. To 2.5 pounds each of lard and castrated boar's butter, add 14 oz. of turpentine oil, 6 oz of white beeswax liquefied over a slow fire; then add 1 oz of precipitated red mercury, 2 ounces each of common dried salt and corrosive mercury sublimate, and a sufficient quantity of sap of the limonium plant and spirits of vinegar for forming the ointment. See Urbano Galeotti *Dissertation upon the diseases, which are treated in the royal hospital of St. Eusebius with the remedies usually used in the same place.* Florence 1771.

~~~~~~~~~~

Elephantiasis

Elephantiasis is lepra predominantly affecting the feet.[1]

Signs. On the affected foot, the little bones of the phalanges gradually swell, expanding the skin and flesh in a surprising manner; the toes fatten and finally liquefy like wax, from which a hemorrhage occurs due to a most trivial cause, spontaneously and quickly stopping again. The malady creeps all the way up to the femur, causing contracture of the joints.

At the same time, the adipose tissue and skin settle slowly into folds and wrinkles in such a way that it completely resembles the appearance of the foot of the elephant. Finally, with the legs having been deformed and the digits of the hands swollen around the joints, they successively loosen and drop off; thenceforth without pain the ulcers first lay waste to the face and then the fleshy parts with an intolerable stench.

In such an amputated leg, the *anatomist* detects no traces of the external periosteum and bone marrow, nor any cavities of the bones. Almost no blood vessels or lymphatic vessels are observed in the internal parts, and those in the wrinkled skin are varicose and nearly empty; both bones within the legs and the bones of the feet have joined together as if into one, and the interosseous artery has been destroyed.
~~~~~~~~~~

Prognosis. Morbus incipiens subinde curatur, morbus autem inveteratus, insanabilis est.

Curatio morbi incipientis tentatar balneis sulphureis, quibus cicuta, helleborus albus & globuli martiales adduntur. Dein plurima loca recentibus foliis boni Henrici obtegantur, etiam vesicatoria, & lotio partium cum spiritu vini aquoso, sale tartari & spiritu salis ammoniaci in hunc finem laudantur.

Interne purgantia, aquae martiales, juscula viperina, fumaria, sarsaparilla, saponaria, chaerophyllum, agrimonia, radix dulcamarae, lapathum acutum, cortex Winteranus, cortex radicis sassafras & peruvianus[2] laudantur, nec non antimonium crudum, atque tinctura cantharidum.[3]

[1] Cel. Schilling de lepra. Lugd. Bat. 1778

[2] *Artzneykundige Abhandlungen von dem Collegio der Aerzte in London.* 1. B. 18. S.

[3] Murray *de vermibus in lepra obviis, juncta leprosi historia.*

Prognosis. The incipient disease can be cured from time to time; however, the advanced disease is incurable.

The treatment of the incipient disease should be attempted with sulfur baths to which hemlock, white hellebore, and mars balls are added. Then most places should be covered over with fresh leaves of the good-king-henry; also lauded for this purpose are vesicatories, washing of regions with a watery spirit of wine, salt of tartar, and a spirit of ammonia salts.

Internally purgings, martial waters, viper broth, fumaria, sarsaparilla, saponaria, chaerophyllum, agrimony, bittersweet root, lapathum acutum, Winteran bark, bark of root of sassafras, and Peruvian bark[2] are touted, and also crude antimony, as well as tincture of cantharides.[3]

[1] Celebrated G. W. Schilling. *Commentaries on Leprosy*. Leiden, 1778.

[2] *Medical Treatises of the College of Physicians in London*. Book 1, p. 18.

[3] Joannes Murray. *About worms encountered in leprosy, with the story of a leper attached.*

CLASSIS VI. CRUSTAE

Sunt cuticulae mutationes in corpus siccum, emortuum, crassiusculum, a cute deciduum vel ei adhaerens.

Nascuntur ex solidis & fluidis cum glutine morboso exsiccatis.

Species crustarum sunt:

Crusta

Est corpus emortuum, siccum, fusco nigrum, a cute sine suppuratione deciduum, solam epidermidem afficiens.

Species crustarum sunt:

1. **Crusta ulcerum**, ex ulcere male sanato saepe gluten exsudat, quod locum ulceris tali crusta obtegit.

2. **Crusta scabiosa**, in scabie simplici tenues, & glabrae, in putrida autem crassae oriuntur tales crustae, quae virides atque pillosae sunt, sua sponte decidunt.

3. **Crusta variolosa**. Exsiccatae variolae in crustas abeunt, vel sua sponte deciduas, vel ab aegrotis decerpendas.

4. **Crusta cancrosa**, quae cancrum nervosum subinde ad digiti crassitiem comitatur. Unguento mercuriali emollitur.

5. **Crustae leprosae**. V. *Lepra.*

Curatio crustarum exigit ut crustae lacte emolliantur, & dein deglubantur.

CLASS VI. CRUSTS

Crusts result when the epidermis changes into a dry, dead, thick substance, falling off from the skin or sticking to it.

They arise from solids and liquids dried up into a diseased glue.

The types of crusts are:

Crusta

Crusta is a dead, dry, brownish-black substance, falling from the skin without suppuration, affecting only the epidermis.

The species of crust are:

1. **Crusta ulcerum** [crust of ulcer]. From the glue which often exudes over a poorly healed ulcer, a crust forms over the place of the ulcer.

2. **Crusta scabiosa** [scabious crust], in simple scabies, the crusts are thin and smooth; in putrid scabies, however, thick crusts arise, which are green and hairy, and spontaneously fall off.

3. **Crusta variolosa** [smallpox crust]. Dried pox turn into crusts that either spontaneously fall off or are picked off by the affected person.

4. **Crusta cancrosa** [cancerous crust], crusts that accompany vigorous cancer, occasionally the thickness of a digit. It is softened with mercurial unguent.

5. **Crustae leprosae** [leprous crust]. See *Lepra*.

The treatment of crusts requires that the crusts be softened with milk, and then peeled off.

~~~~~~~~~~
~~~~~~~~~~

Eschara

Est corpus subhumidum, fuscum vel nigrum, quod ipsam cutem afficit, & hinc ab ea sine suppuratione non separandum.

Ignis, fulmen, lapis causticus, carbunculus & gangraena sicca cutem adeo in escharam mutare valent.

Curatio exigit pinguia & emollientia, subinde scarificationem, ut ope suppurationis natura facilius escharam a partibus sanis separare possit.

~~~~~~~~~~

Achores seu Scabies Capitis

Format ulcera crustosa, humida, in capillata capitis parte.[1]

Species huius scabiei sunt:

1. **Scabies capitis simplex**. Incipit densissimis granulis ac si ex cute grana milii prominerent, haec granula rumpuntur, & exsudans gluten in toto capillitio ulcera crustosa format; crustae hae sunt ubique foraminosae, ac si tineis essent erosae. Hinc haec scabies capitis etiam *tinea benigna* dicitur. Humiditate scabies capitis a tinea vera differt.

2. **Scabies capitis favosa**. Format ulcera, quae ob foramella ampliora alveolis favi, melle albido turgidis, similia sunt. Incipit vesiculis purulentis, in capillitio sine praevia inflammatione ortis, quae sponte vel levi digitorum pressione crepant, & pultem albidoflavescentem fundunt, atque exsiccatae squammas gryseas relinquunt.

3. **Scabies capitis ficosa**. Si ulcera capillitii in foveolis suis purulentis granula flava, qualia in ficu discissa semina sunt, habent, ficosa vocatur scabies.

4. **Scabies capitis lupina**. Exhibet ulcera sicca, quae marginata sunt squammis callosis, seu lupiorum aut cicerum instar capitata & incrassata.
~~~~~~~~~~

Eschara [eschar]

Eschar is a slightly moist, dark or black substance that affects the skin itself and hence cannot be separated from the skin without suppuration.

Fire, lightning, lapis causticus, carbuncle, and dry gangrene are strong enough to change the skin into an eschar.

The treatment requires greases and emollients, then scarification, so that with the help of suppuration, nature is able to separate the eschar more easily from the healthy part.

~~~~~~~~~~

Achores seu Scabies Capitis [tinea capitis]

Achores or scabies capitis are crusty, wet ulcers that form on the hairy part of the head.[1]

The species of this scabies are:

1. **Scabies capitis simplex** [simple scabies of the head, tinea capitis]. It begins with very dense granules, and if indeed the millet grains project from the skin, these granules rupture, and the exuding glue forms crusty ulcers over the entire scalp; these crusts are everywhere full of holes, as if they had been eroded by worms. Hence, this scabies capitis is also called *tinea benigna*. Because of moisture, scabies capitis is different from true scabies.

2. **Scabies capitis favosa** [favus-type tinea capitis]. It forms ulcers that are similar to a honeycomb with enlarged cavities swollen with white honey. It begins with purulent vesicles, arising in the scalp without preceding inflammation. These ulcers break open spontaneously or with light pressure of the fingers and pour out a yellow-white mush which leaves behind gray scales when it dries out.

3. **Scabies capitis ficosa** [fig-like scabies of the head, tinea capitis]. If the ulcers of the scalp have yellow granules in their purulent openings, which are like the seeds in a cut-open fig, the scabies is called *ficosa*.

4. **Scabies capitis lupina** [lupin-like scabies of the head, tinea capitis]. It exhibits dry ulcers, which are marginated with scaly calluses forming a head and thickened, with the appearance either of lupin seeds or chickpeas.
~~~~~~~~~~

Causa proxima est mucus animalis acescens ac rancidulus.[2]

Causae remotae sunt aetas tenera praesertim ablactata, rarius aetas adulta. Diaeta prava, labes haereditaria, metastasis humoris retenti, menstruatio suppressa.

Prognosis. Scabies capitis est critica evacuatio humoris acrimoniosi, qui per glandulas capillitii excernitur. Hinc est morbus infantibus salubris, sed neglectus & diu durans cranii ossa inficit, & tunc difficillime sanatur.

Scabies haecce pruritu, dolore & ingenti foetore infantes molestat, pallorem faciei, noctes insomnes, maciem quandoque cum febre hectica causat, & ob pectinationis vel defectum, vel difficultatem ingens pediculorum copia nascitur. Scabiei excretio frigore vel exsiccantibus *suppressa* pessimos oculorum, cerebri aut pulmonum morbos procreat, ut febrem, caecitatem, ophthalmiam, epilepsiam, convulsionem, glandularum colli intumescentias, tussim, phtysim, anasarcam, hydropem cerebri, apoplexiam.

Curatio exigit:

1. *tonsuram* capillitii, & *pectinationem* cum scopula setacea.

2. *Lotionem* capillitii cum aqua furfurum vel hordei cum melle, vel cataplasma ex farina avenae cum aqua & butyro, folia boni Henrici vel brassicae crispae viridis capiti applicata, nasturtii succum cum pinguedine anseris, camphoram lacte solutam.

3. *Purgantia* saepius repetita.

4. *Decocta purificantia* ex bardana vel lapatho, & fumaria. Aquas acidulas martiales, cort. peruvi.

5. Caput semper mitris & linteis calidum fervetur, *Diaeta* observetur salubris.

Scabies capitis *retropulsa* exigit sinapismum, vel vesicatorium abraso capiti imponendum, ut revocetur scabies, vel denique novam infectionem ope applicatae mitrae scabiosae.

[1] D. Mihr *diss. de achoribus.* Budae 1783

[2] Cel. Lorry *de m. cut.* p. 439.

~~~~~~~~~~
~~~~~~~~~~

The proximate cause is a souring and rancid animal mucus.[2]

The remote causes are young age, especially after being weaned from the breast; it is rarer in adults with the causes being an unbalanced diet; hereditary defect; spreading of retained humor; and suppressed menstruation.

Prognosis. Scabies capitis is a critical evacuation of acrid humor, which is excreted through the glands of the scalp. Hence it is a beneficial disease for infants, but when neglected and long-lasting, it infects the bones of the skull, and then it is cured with very great difficulty.

This scabies troubles infants with itching, pain, and intense malodor; it causes pallor of the face, nocturnal insomnia, emaciation sometimes with hectic fever, and from either failure or difficulty with combing, a prodigious amount of lice is born. The excretion of scabies that is *suppressed* by cold or drying generates very bad diseases of the eyes, brain, or lungs, such as fever, blindness, ophthalmia, epilepsy, convulsion, swelling of the glands of the neck, cough, phthisis, anasarca, hydrops of the brain, and apoplexy.

The treatment requires:

1. Cutting the hair and combing it with a bristly brush.

2. Washing the scalp with bran or barley water with honey, or a cataplasm of wild oat flour with water and butter, leaves of the good-king-henry or curly green cabbage applied to the scalp, nasturtium juice with goose fat, camphor dissolved in milk.

3. *Purging* repeated rather often.

4. *Purifying decoction* from burdock root or lapathum and fumaria, and Peruvian bark in slightly acidic martial water.

5. The head should always be kept warm with turbans and linen; a healthy regimen should be observed.

Retrograde scabies capitis requires that a mustard plaster or a vesicatory be placed on the shaved scalp, in order that the scabies—or even a new infection—might be withdrawn by the power of a turban applied for scabies.

[1] Ferdinand Joseph Muehr. *Dissertation on Achor.* Budae, 1783.

[2] Anne-Charles Lorry. *Treatise on Diseases of the Skin*, 1777. p. 439.

~~~~~~~~~~
~~~~~~~~~~

Crusta Capitis Neunatorum

Est crusta sicca, & crassa, quae in infantibus brevi post partum verticem & sinciput tegere, & saepe medium per annum durare solet.

Curatio. Praeter purificationem cum scopula setacea nihil tentetur, nam suo tempore sponte evanescit.

~~~~~~~~~~

Crusta Lactea

Est eruptio crustarum in genis vel alio faciei loco.

1. **Crusta lactea infantum.**[1] Erumpunt in genis pustulae latae vel acutae, humore limpido, glutinoso plenae, quibus ruptis liquor effluit glutinosus, tenax, cuti adhaerens, qui crustam flavo-rubram efficit. Crusta ipsa saepe finditur, eque fissuris humor glutinosus, crustae crassitiem & duritiem augens, effunditur. Cutis ipsa adfecta dura redditur & partes subjectae intumescunt.

Tumidae simul sunt glandulae jugulares, raro parotides. Aliquando crustae ejusmodi serpunt ad auriculas, aut e mento erumpunt, imo quandoque frontem occupant & totam faciem, exceptis palpebris, larva tegunt. Quandoque ophthalmia vel otorrhaea simul contingit. Quandoque ad reliquum corpus, ut collum, pectus, abdomen, nates & extremitates a facie transeunt.

Aetas. Infantibus lactentibus magis quam ablactatis, semestribus magis, quam qui dentibus jam gaudent, familiaris est morbus. Interdum vero etiam serius incipit morbus atque ultra dentium eruptionem perstat, interdum recurrit.

Causa proxima acris mucus metastatice ad faciem depositus esse videtur. Non videtur morbus esse haereditarius, neque aliis infantibus contagiosus.[2] Infantes enim reliqui innocue cum crustosis in eodem lecto dormivisse fuere visi, atque unus e pluribus infantibus ab eadem matre lactatis morbo solum corripitur.
~~~~~~~~~~

Crusta Capitis Neunatorum [cradle cap]

Crusta capitis neonatorum is a dry, thick crust, which in infants shortly after birth covers the crown of the head and forehead, commonly lasting for half a year.

Treatment. Nothing should be tried except cleaning with a bristle brush, for it spontaneously disappears in its own time.

~~~~~~~~~~

Crusta Lactea [milky crust]

Crusta lactea is an eruption of crust on the cheeks or other parts of the face.

1. **Crusta lactea infantum** [infantile milky crust].[1] Broad or pointed pustules erupt on the cheeks, full of a clear, glutinous humor; after bursting, a viscous fluid flows out, tenacious, clinging to the skin, which produces a yellow-red crust. The crust itself is often cracked, and from the fissures the glutinous humor, increasing the thickness and hardness of the crust, is poured out. The skin itself is affected and becomes hard, and the underlying parts become swollen.

The jugular glands are swollen at the same time, but rarely the parotid glands. Sometimes crusts of this kind spread to the external ears, or break out from the chin; indeed, as often as not they take over the forehead and cover the whole face—except the eyelids—with a horrific mask. Sometimes ophthalmia or otorrhea happens at the same time. Sometimes they cross over from the face to the rest of the body, such as the neck, chest, abdomen, buttocks, and extremities.

Age. The disease is more common in lactating infants than it is in weaned ones, in those older than six months, or in those who are already showing teeth. Occasionally, however, the disease begins even later and persists until after the teeth erupt; sometimes it recurs.

The proximate cause seems to be an acrid mucus deposited metastatically to the face. The disease does not seem to be hereditary, nor contagious to other infants.[2] For I have seen infants who had been sleeping in the same bed with those covered in crusts remain unharmed; I have also seen only one of many infants having been nursed by the same mother corrupted by the disease.
~~~~~~~~~~

Exitus. Diuturnus est morbus, qui infantibus quietem & alacritatem detrahit. Ingentem quandoque excitat pruritum, unde infantum fletus, pervigilium, pavor in somno, & alvus tarda: solvitur morbus per urinam tetri odoris, qualem urina fellis spargit.

Nihil mali a morbo remansisse patet, si facies post sanationem mollis.

Sustinuisse hominem v. g. nutricem in sua infantia hunc morbum conjicimus, si cutis faciei solito magis glabra, & exesa circa genas tenui lanugine polita & splendens est, reliqua vero faciei cutis albida magis est, si erubescens non roseo sed coccineo seu scarlatinoso rubore suffunditur, sed per latas maculas interposita albedine distinguitur.

Curatio exigit, ut purgatis primis viis infanti quotidie lac, in quo pugillus unus jaceae seu violae tricoloris recentis incoquatur, detur. Sic intra 3 vel 4 septimanas hic morbus tuto curatur.

Alii angelicam, levisticum, imperatoriam, aurum in decocto laudant. Alii fuliginem ad gr. iv in syrupo cichorei.[3]

Externe evitentur medicamenta plumbata, exsiccantia & oleosa. Facies cum decocto quodam in quo bilis bubula solvitur quotidie lavetur. Cremor lactis acidulus crustis illinitus pulchre sopit pruritum. Nutrix bonam servet diaetam & iisdem ut infans utatur medicamentis.

Nihil mali a morbo remansisse patet, si facies post delapsum crustarum mollis nec supra pinguedinem tumida, cutis tenuis, non dura vel coriacea aut squammulis aspera & urina sana.

2. **Crusta lactea infantum larvata**. Ante crustae lactea eruptionem ophthalmia, obstructio glandularum, lippitudo, otorrhaea, tabes infantes, afficit.

Nisi quid crustosi in facie se ostendat, lactentis facies crassior est, quam a sola pinguedine exspectes, buccae tumidae, rotundae. Cutis genarum profunde rubra, cutis subjecta dura in pliculas trahi se non sinit, cuticula digito

Resolution. The disease is long-lasting, and it takes away rest and liveliness from the infants. Sometimes it causes prodigious itching, from which the weeping infant cries and remains restless through the night. There is trembling during sleep and sluggish bowels. The disease is released through the urine with a foul odor, such as the urine a cat sprays.

It is evident that no harm has remained from the disease if the face is soft after healing.

We infer that a person has experienced this disease—for example, the nurse in her own infancy—if the skin of the face is more nearly hairless than usual and polished and bright from the thin lanugo being eaten away around the cheeks; if indeed the skin on the remainder of the face is more whitish; and if blushing is suffused not with pink but scarlet or scarlatinous redness. But it is distinguished by the broad spots interposed with the whiteness.

Treatment requires that after the infant's gastrointestinal tract has been purged, milk boiled with one handful of brown knapweed or fresh tricolor violet should be given to the infant every day. Thus, within 3 or 4 weeks, this disease is treated safely.

Some recommend angelica, lovage, or masterwort in a decoction. Others recommend 4 grams of soot in chicory syrup.[3]

Externally, lead-based, drying and oily medicaments should be avoided. The face should be washed daily with a certain decoction in which beef bile is dissolved. Cream of lightly soured milk smeared on the crusts beautifully calms the itch. The wet nurse should maintain a good diet and use the same medication as the baby.

It is evident that no harm has remained from the disease if, after the crusts have separated, the face is soft and not on top of swollen fatness, and the skin is thin, not hard or leathery or with rough scales, and the urine is healthy.

2. **Crusta lactea infantum larvata** [mask-like infantile milky crust]. Before the eruption of the crusta lactea, infants are afflicted with ophthalmia, obstruction of the glands, blepharitis, otorrhea, and wasting.

If something crusty does not show itself on the face, the face of the suckling infant is thicker than you would expect from fatness alone, the cheeks swollen and rounded. The skin of the cheeks is profoundly red; the underlying,

explorata aspera & elevatis minimis squammulis hirta. Frictio partis ab infante tentatur, urina foetida quandoque.

Non satis egressis papulis efficit materia crustae lacteae latens infarctum glandularum meseraicarum, unde tympanites, bulimia, tabes. Repressis autem papulis crustosis morbi glandularum, tussis, asthma, tabes saepe oriuntur.

Curatio exigit, ut purgatis primis viis decoctum violae tricoloris vel pulvis ejusdem detur.

3. **Crusta lactea puerperarum.**[4] In puerperis quandoque a metastasi lactea in genis, mento, palpebris, imo & oculo pustulae citra erysipelas, pure lacteo turgentes, summe prurientes, quae horridae visui, ruborem cuti conciliant, imo crustae cute magis depressae apparent cum odore gravi foetido. Hae crustae non raro abeunt & redeunt, siphilidem simulant, at a dato mercurio summa oriuntur mala.

Curatio. Salus a cura metastasibus congrua, ut a purgantibus, decocto stipitum dulcamarae & arcano duplicato.

[1] Cel. Strack *de crusta lactea infantum ejusdemque specifico remedio diss. Francof. ad Moenum*, 1779.

[2] Anonimi alicujus authoris *Ausführliche Abhandlung von Sägesprüngen einer bekannten Kinderkrankheit.* Nürnberg. 1779

[3] L. c. p. 55.

[4] Cel. Lorry *de morbis cutaneis* p. 283.

~~~~~~~~~~

Tinea

Noscitur crustis viridescentibus, siccis & pertinacibus, quae capillitium atque marginem frontalem occupant.[1]
~~~~~~~~~~

hardened skin does not permit itself to be drawn into small folds, the cuticle explored with the finger feels rough on account of very small raised scales. Rubbing of the area might be attempted by the infant. The urine is sometimes fetid.

The hidden material within the not-quite-egressed papules of crusta lactea causes infarction of the mesenteric glands, leading to abdominal distention, bulimia, and wasting. However, diseases of the glands, cough, asthma, and wasting often arise from repressed crusty papules.

The treatment requires that after a purging of the GI tract, a decoction of tricolor violet or powder of the same be given.

3. **Crusta lactea puerperarum** [postpartum milky crust].[4] In the neonatal period there are sometimes pustules just short of erysipelas from metastasis of milk on the cheeks, chin, eyelids, diaper area, and the eye. These pustules, swelling with milky pus, have extreme itching and are horrible in appearance, bringing redness to the skin; finally, additional depressed crusts appear on the skin with a severely fetid odor. These crusts occasionally go away and return; they simulate syphilis, but if mercury is given, the greatest evils arise.

Treatment. Healing for the metastasis comes with suitable attention, such as purgings with a decoction of bittersweet root and potassium sulfate.

[1] Carl Strack. *Dissertation on the milky crust of infants and its specific remedy, Frankfurt am Main*, 1779.

[2] Anonymous author. *Detailed treatise on the prognosis of a well-known childhood disease.* Nuremberg. 1779

[3] Ibid, p. 55.

[4] The celebrated Anne-Charles Lorry. *Treatise on Diseases of the Skin*, 1777. p. 283.

~~~~~~~~~~

Tinea

Tinea is known by greenish, dry, and tenacious crusts that occur on the scalp and the margin of the forehead.[1]
~~~~~~~~~~

Tinea *species* sunt:

1. **Tinea vera seu crustosa** format crustas viridescentes, cineritias vel nigricantes. Peculiare miasma huius morbi causa esse videtur.

Curatio exigit

1. *purgantia* mercurialia saepius repetita:

2. Decocta *purificantia*, medicamenta *mercurialia* & *sulphurea*. Cicuta,[2] ledum palustre, lapatum acutum, specifica censentur.

Externe 1. Capilli sunt *abscindendi*.

2. Crustae *unguento juniperino*, vel cicuta in lacte cocta emolliantur.

3. Dein capilli & crustae *emplastro picato* eradicentur.

4. Caput saepius *lotione helleborata*, vel solutione salina, ut ex sale alcalino, vel ex sale tartari vel sedo acri contuso, vel spiritu salis unguento mixto, vel unguento sulphuris cum succo citri, abluatur.

2. **Tinea venerea**. Praeter luis venereae signa adsunt crustae albae circa tempora & frontem, & in malo inveterato maculae & pustulae venereae frontis, atque herpes farinaceus aurium.

Curatur haec tinea interno usu mercurii.

Externe unguentum cum praecipitato rubro prudenter adhibeatur.

In malo inveterato lotionem cum solutione sublimati, vel penicillationem crustarum cum aqua caustica pro condilomatibus utilem deprehendi.

[1] D. Steger *diss. de Tinea*. Budae 1782.

[2] Ill. Stoerck *libel. de cicuta* pag. 173. & Cel. Stoelleri *Beobachtungen* p. 139. externo & interno usu cicutae tineam curarunt.

The *species* of tinea are:

1. **Tinea vera (or crustose)** [true tinea or crusty tinea], forms greenish, ashy-gray, or blackish crusts. The cause of this disease seems to be a particular miasma.

Treatment requires:

1. Oft-repeated *purging* with mercurials.
2. *Purifying decoctions*, medicaments of *mercury* and *sulfurous*. Hemlock,[2] wild rosemary, lapathum acutum, are to be considered specifically.

Externally 1. The hair *must be cut off.*

2. The crusts should be softened with *ointment of juniper* or hemlock cooked in milk.
3. Then the hair and crusts are to be uprooted with a *tarry plaster.*
4. The head should be washed fairly often with *hellebore lotion*; or saline solution as from alkaline salt or from salt of tartar; or crushed bitter houseleek, or an ointment mixed with the spirit of salt, or with an ointment of sulfur with citrus juice.

2. **Tinea venerea** [venereal tinea]. In addition to the signs of venereal lues, white crusts form around the temples and forehead; and in the chronically ill, venereal macules and pustules are present on the forehead, as are meal-like herpes on the ears.

This tinea is treated with internal use of mercury.

Externally, ointment with red precipitate should be used prudently.

In the chronically ill, I found useful for condylomas a washing with sublimate solution, or brushing of the crusts with caustic water.

[1] Joachim Paulus Steger. *Dissertation on Tinea.* Budae 1782.

[2] Illustrious Anthony Störck. *An Essay on the Medicinal Nature of Hemlock. In two parts. To Which is Annexed, a Necessary Supplement on the Subject.* p. 173 & Celebrated Friedrich Christian Stoeller *Observations and experiences from internal and external healing.* p. 139. They are curing tinea with the external and internal use of hemlock.

Mentagra

Est peculiaris scabies circa mentum, quae in crustas abit.

Species sunt:

1. **Mentagra venerea**. Ingentem numerum talium crustarum, gluten viscidum exsudantium bis, in magna copia venereorum vidi. Praeter usum internum mercurii pars affecta aliquoties de die aqua phagaedenica, vel solutione sublimati vel lacte mercuriali ablui debet, unguentum mercuriale de nocte imponatur. His remediis non juvantibus illinantur crustae aqua caustica ad condylomata.

2. **Mentagra leprosa** est lepra, mentum & faciem afficiens. *Curatur* ut *lepra.*

3. **Mentagra infantum**. V. *Crusta lactea* in mento.

4. **Mentagra plinii**. Fuit impetigo in mento, quae Romae quondam contagiosa fuit. Vide *Impetigo.*

~~~~~~~~~~

Malum Mortuum

Est pustula, quae in crustam fuscam, latam & crassam cum quadam insensilitate & turpi aspectu, abit.

In coxis & tibiis frequenter observatur, rarius in facie.

Subinde unica est in toto corpore, subinde plures, sed distantissimae observantur. Hae crustae sunt siccae sine dolore, fixae, pertinacissimae, vix pruriginosae. Crustis elapsis cutis infra est granulosa sed non exulceratur.

Sanatur ut tinea per dropacismum V. *tineam.*

~~~~~~~~~~

Mentagra

Mentagra is a particular scabies around the chin, which turns into crusts.

The species are:

1. **Mentagra venerea** [venereal mentagra]. On two occasions, I have seen in a great multitude of venereals an enormous number of such crusts, exuding a viscous glue. In addition to the internal use of mercury, the affected part should be washed several times a day with phagadenic water, or with a solution of sublimate or mercurial milk, a mercurial ointment should be applied at night. When these remedies are not helpful, the crusts should be smeared with caustic water as for condylomata.

2. **Mentagra leprosa** [leprous mentagra] is lepra affecting the chin and face. It is treated as *lepra.*

3. **Mentagra infantum** [infantile mentagra]. See *crusta lactea* on the chin.

4. **Mentagra plinii** [mentagra of Pliny] was impetigo on the chin, which was once contagious in Rome. See *impetigo.*

~~~~~~~~~

Malum Mortuum [deadly evil, ecthyma]

Malum mortuum is a pustule that turns into a dark, wide, and thick crust with a certain numbness and unsightly aspect.

It is frequently observed on the hips and shins, more rarely on the face.

Sometimes there is only one on the entire body, sometimes more, but they are observed very far apart. These crusts are dry, painless, fixed, very stubborn, but scarcely itchy. The skin under the released crusts is grainy but not ulcerated.

It is healed as tinea through a pitch depilatory. See *tinea.*

~~~~~~~~~

Exanthema Labiale

Est efflorescentia vesicularum, quae in labiis erumpunt & cito in parvas crustas abeunt.

Febres intermittentes saepe hac crisi terminantur.

Curatio praeter interna remedia diluentia nihil exigit.

Exanthema Subaxillare

Est efflorescentia vesicularum, quae in cavo subaxillari uno vel utroque erumpunt, magnam copiam humoris viscidi saepe excernunt & in crustas tenues ebeant.

Eruptio tempore aestivo frequenter contingit.

Curatio exigit diligentem ablutionem cum aqua calida, & interna remedia diluentia: jusculum cum chaerophyllo & fumaria profuit.

Exanthema Labiale [herpes labialis]

Exanthema labiale is a blossoming of vesicles that erupt on the lips and quickly turn into small crusts.

Intermittent fevers often end at this point.

Treatment requires nothing besides internal cleansing remedies.

Exanthema Subaxillare [bullous impetigo]

Exanthema subaxillare is a blossoming of vesicles that erupt in the vault of one or both underarms, often discharging a copious amount of viscous humor, and evolve into thin crusts.

It frequently occurs in the summertime.

The treatment requires diligent washing with hot water and internal cleansing remedies: broth with chaerophyllum and fumaria has been of benefit.

CLASSIS VII. SQUAMMAE

Haec classis continet morbos cutaneos, in quibus cuticula tota vel sub forma squammarum vel furfurum a cute secedit.

Species hujus classis sunt:

~~~~~~~~~~

Furfuratio

Est epidermidis secessus sub forma *furfurum.*

Furfuratio est raro morbus per se, sed utplurimum symptoma porriginis, herpetis.

Curatio hinc juxta morbum, a quo oritur, institui debet.

~~~~~~~~~~

Desquammatio

Est epidermidis secessus sub forma *squammarum.*

Hic morbus etiam symptoma est impetiginis, vel ichtyosis [*sic*], hinc ut hi morbi curatur.

Exuvia Epidermidis

Est cuticulae secessus a cute sub forma magnarum laminarum. Causae, quae epidermidem a cute in latis portionibus solvunt, sunt 1. inflammatio erysipelacea. 2. Calor aquae ebullientis, aut solis. 3. Maceratio cutis in aqua. 4. Putredo gangraenosa. 5. Vesicatorium aut aliud acre cuti impositum. 6. Acrimonia sub epidermidem deposita, ut in quibusdam febribus & ab esu delphini contingit.

Curatio externa exigit, ut pinguia, butyrum simplex aut ex fructu cacao applicetur, sic facile & sua sponte renascitur epidermis.

CLASS VII. SCALES

This class contains skin diseases in which the whole cuticle separates from the skin in either the form of scales or dandruff.

The species of this class are:

~~~~~~~~~~

Furfuratio [dandruff]

Furfuratio is the separation of the epidermis in the form of *dandruff.*

Furfuratio is rarely a disease per se, but almost always symptomatic of porrigo and herpes.

Thus, treatment should be started according to the illness from which it originates.

~~~~~~~~~~

Desquammatio [desquamation]

Desquamation is the separation of the epidermis in the form of scales.

This disease is also a symptom of impetigo or ichthyosis; hence, it is treated as these diseases are treated.

Exuvia Epidermidis [exfoliation]

Exuvia epidermidis is the separation of the cuticle in the form of large sheets. The causes that split the epidermis from the skin in wide portions are: 1. erysipelatous inflammation, 2. heat from boiling water or sun, 3. maceration of the skin in water, 4. putrefied gangrene, 5. a vesicatory or other harsh substance applied to the skin, 6. corrosive substance deposited under the epidermis, as happens in certain fevers or from eating dolphin.

External treatment requires that lard, simple butter or butter from cacao fruit be applied, so that the epidermis is easily and spontaneously reborn.

Exuvia epidermidis & Cutis a raphania. Non solum epidermis sed & ipsa vera cutis hinc inde secedit, adeo ut nudi musculi & tendines videri possint.[1] *Medela* exigit, ut externe unguentum saturninum applicetur.

[1] Cel. Taube *Geschichte der Kriebel - Krankheit.* 1782. *Göttingen* p. 153.

~~~~~~~~~~

Porrigo

Est morbus, in quo in capillata capitis parte rimae siccae & callosae oriuntur, quae perpetuo scatent furfure albescente inter pectinandum deciduo.

Species sunt:

1. **Porrigo furfuracea**, quam mox descripsi.

2. **Porrigo lupina**, quae squammas instar cicerum format. Vide Scabies capitis lupina.

3. **Porrigo farinosa seu spuria**, est congeries materiei unguinosae pulverulentae, quae ob pectinationis defectum in capite cumulatur, & crustam sordidam, atque faetidam, sub pectine farinae crassae forma delabentem, constituit.

Materies haec farinosa vel furfuracea humor sebaceus glandularum capitis esse videtur. Sub his sordibus copiosa proles pediculorum tuta hospitatur.

Curatio exigit diligentem & frequentem pectinationem. Porrigo autem *vera* seu *furfuracea*, ut *scabies capitis*, curatur.

~~~~~~~~~~

Exuvia epidermidis et cutis a raphania [exfoliation of epidermis and skin from the wild radish]. Not only the epidermis, but also the true skin itself separates here and there, to such a degree that the bare muscles and tendons can be seen.[1] Healing requires that saturnine ointment be applied externally.

[1] Celebrated Johann Taube *The History of Crawly Disease*. Gottingen, 1782. p. 153.

~~~~~~~~~~

Porrigo [seborrheic dermatitis]

Porrigo is a disease in which dry and calloused cracks arise on the hairy part of the head, from which abundant whitish branny scales constantly fall out while being combed.

The species are:

1. **Porrigo furfuracea** [furfuraceous porrigo, seborrheic dermatitis], which I have just described.

2. **Porrigo lupina** [lupin-like porrigo, seborrheic dermatitis], which forms squames with the appearance of chickpeas. See scabies capitis lupina.

3. **Porrigo farinosa or spuria** [farina-like or false porrigo, seborrheic dermatitis] is an accumulation of greasy, powdery material that is built up on the head from failure to comb and forms a dirty crust and also a foul odor; it descends under the comb with the appearance of a thick flour.

This floury or branny matter seems to be the sebaceous humor of the glands of the head. A great number of the offspring of lice are harbored safely under this filth.

Treatment requires careful and frequent combing. Indeed, *true* or *furfuraceous* porrigo is treated as *scabies of the head.*

~~~~~~~~~~

Lichen

Est macula solitaria, rubra, aspera, sicca, admodum pruriens, quae in tenuissimum furfurem solvitur.

Causa est peculiaris acrimonia. *Curatur* ut *impetigo*, cuius levissima esse videtur species. *Externe* saliva jejuna aut solutione sublimati cum sale ammoniaco, aut unguento helleborato vel ex mercurio praecipitato rubro vel albo macula fricati debet.

~~~~~~~~~~

Impetigo

Est morbus, in quo multae maculae rubrae, durae, siccae, prurientes & asperae oriuntur, quae a facie vel collo ortae, totum corpus petunt & vel in furfures vel in tenues squammas resolvuntur. Hinc est *lichen* in toto corpore.

Species sunt:

1. **Impetigo benigna**. Cutis maculae rubentes & prurientes evadunt crassae, durae & tumidae, nec non leviter humescunt, & ex humore albido transsudante squammae fiunt albae, crassitie papyrum tenuissimam aequantes, quae tam digitis aufferri possunt, quam per sudores decidunt, quibus demptis profluit sanguis. Haec impetigo etiam ungues aliquantum destruit. Subinde in capitis cute incipit.

2. **Impetigo maligna**, est illa, quae cutem pessime exulcerat.

3. **Impetigo hereditaria**, quae in infante a parentibus eodem morbo affectis observatur.

4. **Impetigo a contagio**, ut balneo, lecto, osculo contracta. Solis osculis impetigo menti Romae quondam pandemia fuit.[1]

5. **Impetigo senum**, quae ab acrimonia senili in senibus observatur.
~~~~~~~~~~

Lichen

Lichen is a solitary, red, rough, dry, very itchy macule that breaks up into very thin furfuraceous scale.

The cause is a particular acrimony. It is treated as *impetigo*, of which it seems to be the mildest species. Externally, fasting saliva or sublimate solution with ammonium chloride, or hellebore ointment, or ointment from red or white mercury precipitate should be rubbed on the spot.

~~~~~~~~~~

Impetigo

Impetigo is a disease in which many red, firm, dry, itchy, and rough macules arise; having appeared on the face or neck, they attack the entire body and are resolved into either branny scales or thin squames. Hence, impetigo is lichen on the entire body.

The species are:

1. **Impetigo benigna** [benign impetigo, psoriasis]. Reddening and itching macules of the skin become thick, hard, and swollen, and slightly moist; from their white transudating humor arise white scales, equaling the thinnest papyrus in thickness, which can be removed with the fingers, the same as by wiping off sweat; and after the scales have been removed, blood flows. This impetigo even destroys the nails somewhat. From time to time, it extends to the scalp.

2. **Impetigo maligna** [malignant impetigo] is that impetigo which ulcerates the skin very badly.

3. **Impetigo hereditaria** [hereditary impetigo], which is observed in an infant from parents affected by the same disease.

4. **Impetigo a contagio** [impetigo from contagion, impetigo contagiosa], contracted from a bath, bed, or kiss; impetigo of the chin from kisses alone was at one time pandemic in Rome.[1]

5. **Impetigo senum** [senile impetigo] is observed in the elderly from acrimony of old age.
~~~~~~~~~~

6. **Impetigo ab ingestis acribus** ut salis, vini vel aromatum abusu.

7. **Impetigo venerea**, quae a viru venereo.

8. **Impetigo scorbutica** quae, a scorbuto.

9. **Impetigo leprosa**, quae a lepra latente.

10. **Impetigo febrisequa**, quae febres quandoque sequitur. Cortex tentandus.

11. **Impetigo retropulsa**, asthma, caecitatem & alios morbos infert, hinc acrimonia in cutem vesicatoriis est reducenda.

Causa proxima impetiginis est serum acre in cutem depositum. Serum acre redditur victu salso & acri, acrimonia latente venerea, aut scorbutica, aut leprosa. Nam hos in morbos saepe malum erumpit.

Curatio impetiginis benignae tentatur:

1. *Purgantibus*, cicuta, acidulis, succo pomorum acidorum, cort. peruv., sarsaparilla.

2. *Decoctis purificantibus* chamomillae & fumariae.

3. *Solutione* mercurii sublimati.

Externe balnea ex chamomillis vel thermis sulphureis conducunt, laudantur praeterea externe radix lapati aceto macerata, succus ricini contusi, spiritus ligni sancti, sapo venetus cum spiritu vini rectificato, oleum tartari per deliquium, sinapi, medicamenta sulphurata, mercurialia, plumbata, martialia.[2] Efficacissimum vero remedium esse censetur herba antilichenia.[3] In impetigine *scorbutica* & *venerea* simul antidota harum acrimoniarum adhibeantur.

[1] Plinii *Hist. nat.* L. 26. C. I. Cel. Gruner *morb. antiquit.* p. 162. solide monstrat mentagram Plinii impetiginem fuisse.

6. **Impetigo ab ingestis acribus** [impetigo from ingesting bitter substances], which is from the abuse of ingesting acrid substances such as salt, wine, or spices.

7. **Impetigo venerea** [venereal impetigo], which is from a venereal virus.

8. **Impetigo scorbutica** [scorbutic impetigo], which is from scurvy.

9. **Impetigo leprosa** [leprous impetigo], which is from latent lepra.

10. **Impetigo febrisequa** [impetigo after fever], which sometimes follows fevers. Bark ought to be tried.

11. **Impetigo retropulsa** [retrograde impetigo] brings asthma, blindness, and other diseases; hence the acrimony must be reduced in the skin with vesicatory agents.

The proximate cause of impetigo is an acrid serum deposited on the skin. The serum is rendered acrid by a salty and acrid diet, or by a latent venereal, scorbutic, or leprous acrimony. For this affliction often bursts forth into these diseases.

The treatment of impetigo benigna is proven to be:

1. *Purgings* with hemlock, mineral waters, juice of acidic fruits, Peruvian bark, sarsaparilla.

2. *Purifying decoctions* of chamomile and fumaria.

3. *Solution* of sublimated mercury.

Externally, chamomile baths or thermal sulfurous baths are expedient. Also praised for external use is *radix lapati* soaked in vinegar; juice of crushed ricinus, spirit of ligni sancti, Venetian soap with rectified spirit of wine, oleo tartari per deliquium; also mustard, sulfurous, mercurial, lead-based, or martial medications.[2] The most effective remedy is regarded to be an anti-lichen herb.[3] For impetigo scorbutica and venerea, the antidotes of these acrimonies should be applied at the same time.

[1] Pliny the Elder. *Historia naturalis.* Book 26. Chapter 1.
The celebrated Christian Gottfried Gruner. *Diseases of Antiquity.* 1774. p. 162.
They definitively show Pliny's mentagra to have been impetigo.

[2] De his omnibus vide egregiam D. Lupini *diss. de lichene*. Budae 1778.

[3] Cel. Hillary *Beobachtungen uber die Veränderung der Luft auf der Insel Barbados*. p. 430.

~~~~~~~~~~

Ichthyosis

Est morbus, in quo diversae corporis partes teguntur squammis siccis & albidis, successive superincumbentibus, eodem ordine ac modo, quo squammae piscium sibi incumbunt. [1]

Aegroti subinde ut pisces foetent, & in Asia squammae circulo rubro sunt cinctae.

Curatio. Specificum & unicum in hoc morbo remedium est decoctum ex cortice intermedio ulmi.[2]

[1] *Acta Lipsiensia* 1688. & Cel. Sauvages *Nosologia methodica* T. II. p. 572.

[2] Cel. Lettsom *Med. Nachrichten von dem allgemeinen Dispensatorio in Londen. Altenb.* 1777. p. 131.

~~~~~~~~~~

Tyriasis

Est leprae species, in qua cutis a carne subjacente putrida facile detrahi potest.[1]

A scalptura cujusvis partis farina ac furfur excutitur, demum ubique oriuntur maculae alba. Nasus & digiti incrassantur, ut in lepra & omnes pili in toto corpore defluunt.

Causa proxima est virus leprosum cum putredine junctum.

Curatio incipientis morbi ut in lepra est, sed adde internum usum acidi vitrioli.

[1] A serpente *tyro*, qui cutem facile exuit, nomen habet.

~~~~~~~~~~
~~~~~~~~~~

[2] See all of these in Daniel-Martinus Lupini. *Dissertation on Lichen*. Budae. 1778.

[3] Celebrated William Hillary. *Observations on Changes of Atmosphere and the Epidemic Sicknesses connected with the Island of Barbadoes*. Leipzig, 1766. p. 430.

~~~~~~~~~~

Ichthyosis

Ichthyosis is a disease in which various parts of the body are covered in dry, whitish scales, successively overlapping, in the same arrangement and manner in which the scales of fish lean on each other.[1]

Sick persons thus reek of fish, and in Asia, the scales are surrounded by a red circle.

Treatment. The one and only remedy for this disease is a decoction from the intermediate bark of the slippery elm tree.[2]

[1] *Proceedings of Erudition of Leipzig*. 1688. & Celebrated Francois Sauvages *Nosologia methodica* (1768). Book II, p. 572.

[2] The celebrated John Coakley Lettsom. *Medical news from the general dispensary in London*. Altenburg, 1777. p. 131.

~~~~~~~~~~

Tyriasis

Tyriasis is a species of lepra in which the skin can be removed easily from the underlying putrid flesh.[1]

Farina and furfur are also cast off by any scratching at all of this area, eventually leaving white spots everywhere. The nose and fingers are thickened, as in lepra, and all hairs on the entire body fall off.

The proximate cause is a leprous virus associated with rottenness.

The treatment in the beginning of the disease is as in lepra, but add internal use of vitriolic acid.

[1] It takes its name from a *Tyrian* snake, which easily sheds its skin.

~~~~~~~~~~
~~~~~~~~~~

Asperitas Cutis

Est cutis aspera, crassa, fusca vel rubens.

Species sunt:

1. **Asperitas a vento**, facies vento frigido diu exposita redditur aspera, sic etiam fit *a frigore*. Est rusticis & peregrinantibus familiaris.

2. **Asperitas a lixivio vel sapone**, quae in manibus lotricum invenitur. Alcali causticum saponis cutem sic deturpat.

3. **Asperitas ab aetate**. Quo provectioris est homo aetatis, eo crassior fit cutis, praesertim in facie.

Curatio cutis asperae butyro cacao & aliis pinguibus obtinetur. *Cosmetica* raro prosunt praeter bilem bubulam.

Cutis Rugosa

Senium, vel peculiaris laxitas cutis vel consuetudo frontem perpetuo rugandi, faciunt ut haec, praesertim in fronte, in rugas contrahatur.

I. **Rugositas a laxitate** fumo aromatico ex myrrha curari dicitur.

2. **Rugositas leprosa**. Frons in hoc morbo rugosa fit, malum ut morbus, a quo oritur, est incurabile.

3. **Rugositas senilis** est incurabilis.

Asperitas Cutis [rough skin]

The skin is rough, thick, brown, or reddening.

The species are:

1. **Asperitas a vento** [rough skin from the wind]. The face is rendered rough when exposed to a cold wind for a long time; this also happens from the *cold*. It is familiar to country people and travelers.

2. **Asperitas a lixivio or sapone** [rough skin from lye or soap], which is found on the hands of washerwomen. Caustic alkaline soap thus disfigures the skin.

3. **Asperitas ab aetate** [rough skin from old age]. The more advanced the age of a man is, the thicker the skin becomes, especially on the face.

The cure of rough skin is obtained with cocoa butter and other fats. *Cosmetics* rarely help except for beef bile (ox gall).

Cutis Rugosa [wrinkles]

Old age, or a particular laxity of the skin, or the habit of constantly wrinkling the forehead makes the skin, especially on the forehead, contract into wrinkles.

1. **Rugositas a laxitate** [wrinkles from laxity] is said to be cured by aromatic smoke from myrrh.

2. **Rugositas leprosa** [leprous wrinkles]. In this disease, the forehead becomes wrinkled; the malady, as is the disease from which it arises, is incurable.

3. **Rugositas senilis** [senile wrinkles] is incurable.

CLASSIS VIII. CALLOSITATES

Sunt mutationes epidermidis in substantiam albidam, duram, crassam & insensilem.

Huc ergo referuntur sequentia *genera*:

Callus

Est epidermis indurata, crassa & insensilis.

Causa proxima est muci malpighiani major secretio, exsiccatio & induratio. Irritatio secretionem, pressio & aer condensationem faciunt.

Causae remotae sunt diuturnus *attritus*, unde major muci malpighiani secretio, & induratio. Idem ab acore minerali[1] & a calore fervido observatur.[2]

Species sunt:

1. **Callus in palmis manuum**, oritur ab assiduo labore, & tractatione instrumentorum crassorum.

2. **Callus in plantis pedum** accrescit, si pedibus nudis longo tempore incedamus.[3] Dolentissimus evadit talis callus, si rimam seu fissuram contrahit. Optimum remedium in hoc morbo fuit mihi unguentum album camphoratum cum unguento neapolitano mixtum, si calceus simul induatur latior.[4]

3. **Callus fistularum & ulcerum**, est margo callosus, qui ulcera circumdat, oritur vi exsiccante aëris aut turundis multum prementibus.

Curatio. Ablata pressione callus manuum & pedum sua sponte sensim evanescit, aut maceratione in aqua, applicatisque unguentis camphoratis emollitur, vesicatorio, vel phosphoro tollitur.

[1] Spiritu vitrioli aut sulphuris adeo cuticula induratur & incrassatur, ut tales ignem devorare possint. Deslandes *Brem. Magazin* T. I. p. 665.

CLASS VIII. CALLUSES

Calluses are changes of the skin into a whitish, hard, thick, and insensate substance.

To that end, the following genera are described:

Callus

Callus is indurated, thickened, and insensate epidermis.

The proximate cause is greater secretion, drying, and induration of malpighian mucus. Irritation causes secretion; pressure and air cause condensation.

The remote causes are rubbing for a long time, whence comes greater secretion of malpighian mucus and induration. The same is observed from an acidic mineral[1] and from fiery heat.[2]

The species are:

1. **Callus in palmis manuum** [palmar callus] arises from continuous labor and from holding heavy instruments.

2. **Callus in plantis pedum** [plantar callus] grows if we march on bare feet for a long time.[3] Such a callus becomes very painful if it contracts a crack or fissure. The best cure for this disease, as far as I am concerned, has been white camphorated ointment mixed with Neapolitan ointment, if a wider shoe is worn at the same time.[4]

3. **Callus fistularum and ulcerum** [callus of a fistula and ulcer] is a callused margin that surrounds ulcers; it arises from the drying force of air or excessive pressure from a bandage.

Treatment. When the pressure is removed, the callus of the hands and feet gradually disappears on its own, or by soaking in water; it is softened with applied camphorated ointments; or it is removed with a plaster that raises blisters on the skin, or with phosphorus.

[1] With the spirit of vitriol or of sulfur, the skin is hardened and thickened to such a degree that such people can swallow fire. Deslandes, *Bremen Magazine for the Propagation of Science, Arts and Virtue*. Book 1. p. 665.

[2] Frictione & ingenti calore destruitur cuticula, at renascitur alia, primae simillima, sed continuata causa frictionis, calorisve ad primam cuticulam novae aliae laminae callosae perpetuo accedunt, quae demum in adeo crassum corneumque tuber abeunt, ut tales homines prunas ardentes vel ferramenta candentia in manu circumgerere, & fuso metallo demum manus lavare discant. Id *Magnus* Boerhaavius de fabris ferrariis testatur, id *Illustr.* Hallerus in vitrariorum officinis vidit.

[3] A sola calida, arena Aegyptiis soleae non minus durae quam bobus sunt. Ut absque dolore possint ferro calceari; & in siamensim regno super ignitas prunas tuto ingrediuntur. *Illustr.* Halleri *Element. Physiologiae* T. V. p. 58.

[4] Cel. Camper. *Abh. über den besten Schuh.* p. 49.

Cicatrix

Est callus a consolidato vulnere vel ulcere relictus.

Formatur a muco malpighiano, quo vulnera ultimatim conglutinantur.

Cicatrix pulchra vocatur, quae cute, nec elevatior, nec depressior est, ut in vulneribus, acuto instrumento inflictis & apte unitis videre est.

Diversae observantur cicatricum *species*:

1. **Cicatrix elevata**, oritur, si caro ultra vulneris libellam luxurians, exsiccantium vi in cicatricem exsiccetur. Hae cicatrices utplurimum iterum aperiuntur, nisi id apta compressione & roborantibus impediatur.

2. **Cicatrix cava**, contingit, si per suppurationem cutis & membrana adiposa multum consumpta est. Sic vulnera cariosa, spina ventosa, & profundae ambustiones relinquunt cicatrices cavas, quae infundibuli forma ad ossa fere pergunt. Hae cicatrices sunt insanabiles.

3. **Cicatrices a graviditate**. Referunt hae cicatrices in regione hypogastrica abdominis, in inguinibus & interioribus femoris partibus *strias albicantes*, adhuc diu post partum conspicuas, sed cum tempore fere evanescentes.

[2] By friction and great heat the skin is destroyed, but another skin is born very similar to the first. However, with the continuous cause of friction or of heat, other new callus layers are constantly added to the first cuticle, which finally morph into such thick and horn-like swelling that such men carry around burning coals or white-hot iron tools in their hands, and finally they learn to wash their hands with molten metal. The great Boerhaave attests to this concerning the iron workers; the illustrious Haller saw this in the workshops of the glassmakers.

[3] From the hot sand alone, the soles of the Aegyptians' feet are not less hard than oxen's feet so that they are able to be shoed with iron without pain, and in the Siamese kingdom they walk safely on burning coals. The illustrious Haller's *Elements of Physiology*. Book V, p. 58.

[4] Peter Camper. *Treatise on the best form of shoes*. p. 49.

Cicatrix [scar]

Cicatrix is a callus left behind from a thickened wound or ulcer.

It is formed from malpighian mucus, with which wounds are ultimately glued together.

A cicatrix is considered aesthetically pleasing if it is neither more elevated nor more depressed than the skin observed in wounds inflicted with a sharp instrument and aptly brought together.

The different species of cicatrices are:

1. **Cicatrix elevata** [elevated scar, hypertrophic scar] arises if flesh swelling up above the level of the wound is dried into a scar by the force of drying substances. These scars are nearly always opened again unless suitably bound with compression and reinforcement.

2. **Cicatrix cava** [caved scar] happens if through suppuration of the skin, much of the adipose tissue has been consumed. In this way decayed wounds, tuberculous dactylitis, and deep burns leave behind caved scars which, after forming a conduit, proceed almost to the bones. These scars are incurable.

3. **Cicatrices a graviditate** [scars of pregnancy, stretch marks] refer to the scars in the region under the umbilicus, in the inguinal area, and in the region medial to the femoral area. These white striae are still seen for a long time after pregnancy but with time nearly disappear.

4. **Cicatrices variolosa**, quae praesertim in facie a praegressis variolis veris remanere solent.

5. **Cicatrices leprae asturiensis,** quae rosei coloris, infra cutis libellam depressae & lucidae esse solent.

~~~~~~~~~~

Clavus

Est tuberculum callosum, album, rotundum, in digitis vel plantis pedum.[1]

Sed clavorum locus frequentissimus in dorso digiti minimi, quandoque vero in aliis, est: quandoque inter digitos in superficie interna utraque duorum digitorum sibi accumbentium duo clavi inveniuntur.

Species clavorum sunt:

1. **Clavi superficiales**, qui epidermidi & cutis superficiei externae solummodo adhaerent.

2. **Clavi profundi**, qui cuti, tendinibus aut periosteo adhaerent, hinc a pressione cutis dolent. In suo centro *nucleum* durissimum habent, quo eradicato pars affecta non dolet, usque dum novus nucleus efformetur.

Nascuntur clavi a pressione loculi digitorum, hinc familiares sunt illis, qui calceis arctioribus aut latioribus utuntur.

Curatio exigit: 1. Ut clavus pediluvio tepido bene emolliatur, & ut nucleus clavi dein unguibus digitorum vel cultello caute eximatur. 2. Dein clavus cera viridi, vel folio sedi, aceto forti macerato, aut emplastro diachilon vel saponato vel emplastro ad clavos per aliquot septimanas tegatur & a pressione defendatur. Subinde clavus solo emplastro vesicatorio vel tinctura cantharidum auferri potest. Efficacissimum remedium est, si globulus ex unguento de ranis cum mercurio quadruplicato ope emplastri longi & tenuis ad clavum applicetur.[2]

Nimis profunde excisus clavus ingentem totius cruris inflammationem, gangraenam, vel cancrum fungosum vel tetanum causare potest.
~~~~~~~~~~

4. **Cicatrices variolosae** [smallpox scars], which usually remain predominantly on the face from the preceding true variola.

5. **Cicatrices leprae asturiensis** [scars of Asturian lepra], which are usually rose-colored, depressed below the level of the skin, and clear.

~~~~~~~~~~

Clavus [corn]

Clavus, or corn, is a callused white, round nodule on the digits or soles of the feet.[1]

But the most frequent location of corns is the dorsum of the smallest toe; sometimes, however, on others; sometimes two corns are found between the digits of the internal surface of each of two digits lying next to the other.

The species of corns are:

1. **Clavi superficiales** [superficial corn], which adhere only to the epidermis and the external surface of the skin.

2. **Clavi profundi** [deep corn], which adhere to the skin, tendons, or periosteum, hurt because of pressure of the skin on this place. They have a very hard nucleus in their center; after the eradication of the nucleus, the affected part does not hurt until a new nucleus is formed.

Clavi arise from the pressure on a small place of the digits; hence, they are familiar to those who wear shoes too narrow or too wide.

The treatment requires: 1. That the corn be well softened with a warm footbath, and that the core of the clavus should then be carefully removed with the nails of the fingers or with a small knife. 2. Then let the clavus be covered with fresh wax, or leaf of the houseleek soaked in strong vinegar, or with a diachylon plaster or a soapy water plaster, applied to the corns for some weeks, and protected from pressure. Thereupon, the clavus can be removed with the vesicating plaster alone or with a tincture of cantharidin. A very effective remedy is a globule of ointment of frogs along with a fourfold amount of mercury applied to the clavus with the help of a durable and thin plaster.[2]

A clavus cut out too deep can cause vast inflammation of the entire leg, gangrene, a fungating cancer, or tetanus.
~~~~~~~~~~

3. **Clavus in planta pedum**. Quandoque unus, quandoque integra congeries clavorum plurium invenitur. *Salus* a foliis sedi minoris recentis contusis & per noctem in aceto maceratis atque clavis applicatis speranda.[3]

4. **Clavus seu verruca sub ungue**. Unguem elevat, ingentem excitat dolorem, & a minima mole quandoque in ingens & durissimum excrescit cornu. *Medela* exigit, ut unguis pediluvio maceratus ad latus utrumque verruca subungualis incidatur, dein unguis a verrucae elevetur & cornu excidatur.[4]

5. **Clavus ad cristam illi**, hic in feminis a nimis arctis thoracibus, cristas ilii prementibus, oritur.

[1] Rousselot *Toilette des pieds.* & Ill. Richters. *Chirurg.* T. I. p. 428.

[2] Cel. Campers. *Abh. über den besten Schuh.* Wien 1782.

[3] *Celeberrimus* Closius, practicus expertissimus Pestinentis aegrotam, quae jam a longo tempore congeriem 16 vel plurium clavorum sub pollicis majoris haluce gerebat, intra aliquot septimanas hac methodo sanabat.

[4] *Cel.* Camper. l. c. p. 52 & 56.

3. **Clavus in planta pedum** [plantar corn]. Sometimes one, sometimes a whole mass of multiple corns is found. Healthy skin is hoped for by applying to the corns freshly pounded, young houseleek leaves that have been soaked in vinegar overnight.[3]

4. **Clavus seu verruca sub ungue** [subungual corn or wart]. A corn or wart elevates the nail, causing severe pain, and sometimes from a minimal mass, a remarkable and very hard horn grows. The treatment requires that after softening the nail in a footbath, each side of the subungual wart should be cut into, then the nail should be raised from the wart and the horn excised.[4]

5. **Clavus ad cristam illi** [corn on the iliac crest], this arises in women from too tight a corset pressing the iliac crests.

[1] Rousselot *Grooming of the feet.* & Illustrious Richters. *Surgery.* Book 1, p. 428.

[2] Celebrated Peter Camper. *Treatise on the best form of shoes.* Vienna, 1782.

[3] The very celebrated Closius, a most experienced practitioner of Pest, cured a sick person within a few weeks with this method who had already for a long time carried a mass of sixteen or more corns under the big toe.

[4] Celebrated Camper. ibid, pp. 52 & 56.

CLASSIS IX. EXCRESCENTIAE CUTANEAE

Sunt parva tubera, quae ultra cutis libellam prominent.

Hi morbi per succi nutrititii copiosiorem affluxum & adhaesionem fieri videntur.

Genera hujus classis sunt :

Verruca

Est tuberculum durum, scabrum, indolens, ex cute prominens.[1] In facie & manibus, raro in partibus aliis nascuntur.

Causa est raro cognita. An acrimonia verrucosa detur, & an haec sit contagiosa, non adeo clare notum est.

Species verrucarum sunt:

1. **Verruca vulgaris**, quae in basi & apice ejusdem diametri est.

2. **Verruca pensilis seu acrochordon** est verruca, quae ope petioli angustioris cuti adhaeret.

3. **Verruca sessilis seu porrum**, est verruca cuti immersa, seu vix extra cutem prominens.

4. **Verruca carnea seu mollusca** est tuberculum molle, sensile, cuti concolor vel rubens, saepe pilosum. In naso & facie utplurimum invenitur. Videtur admodum magna glandula cutanea quasi esse.

5. **Verruca madida seu myrmecium**, est verruca mollis, nuda, & semper madida.

6. **Verruca gregalis**. Dantur verrucae admodum parvae, quae gregatim in facie vel manibus erumpunt, sed etiam saepe sponte evanescunt.

CLASS IX. CUTANEOUS GROWTHS

Cutaneous growths are small protuberances that protrude above the level of the skin.

These diseases seem to be made from the abundant outflowing and adhesion of nutritional juices.

The genera of this class are:

Verruca [wart]

Verruca is a hard, rough, painless nodule protruding from the skin.[1] It arises on the face and hands, rarely on other parts.

The cause is rarely determined; whether it is produced by a verrucous acrimony or whether it is contagious is not yet clearly known.

The species of verrucae are:

1. **Verruca vulgaris** [common wart], in which the diameter is the same at the base and the apex.
2. **Verruca pensilis** [hanging wart] or acrochordon is a wart that adheres to the skin with the help of a rather narrow stalk.
3. **Verruca sessilis or porrum** [sessile wart or porrum] is a verruca immersed in the skin, or barely protruding above the skin.
4. **Verruca carnea or mollusca** [fleshy wart or mollusca] is a soft, sensitive nodule, reddish or skin-colored, often hairy. It is found most often on the nose and face. It seems very much as if it were a large cutaneous gland.
5. **Verruca madida or myrmecium** [moist wart or myrmecial wart] is a soft, bare, and always wet wart.
6. **Verruca gregalis** [grouped warts, flat warts] is the term given to exceedingly small warts that erupt in groups on the face or hands, but also often spontaneously disappear.

7. **Verruca febrilis**, quae cum febre ut exanthema in toto corpore erumpit. V. *Variolas verrucosas.*

8. **Verruca cancrosa seu maligna**, est verruca livens vel rubens, dolens, varicosa, quae in cancrum abit.[2]

9. **Verrucae venereae**, sunt moris, vel frambaesiis similes, quae in venereorum facie erumpunt, ut aliquoties vidi.

Curatio verrucarum obtinetur:

1. *Ligatura*, quae in verrucis petiolatis ope fili sericei, vel setae equinae peragi potest.

2. *Excisione*, qua verrucae cancrosae curantur.

3. *Causticis*: ut spiritu salis concentrato, aqua forti, oleo camphorae caustico, quibus verrucae mediante penicillo bis de die illini debent.

4. *Inustione*, acus ad candelam excalefacta in verrucam infigitur.

5. *Frictione* verrucae cum *sapone nigro*, vel lacte vel folio ficus, vel cerumine aurium.

6. Applicatione *emplastri vesicatorii*, & tincturae cantharidum.

7. *Remediis sympatheticis.* Sic verruca pomo, vel carne, vel sanguine, ex anguillae capite abscisso stillante, multum fricta, & remediis dein in terram sepultis, evanescere dicitur. Mihi res, saepius tentata, non successit.

Verrucae *gregales* saepe dato purgante, dein asa faetida aliquot septimanis assumpta, sponte evanescunt. Verrucae *venereae*, ut condylomata venerea, curantur.

[1] *Ill.* Richter *Chirurgie* T. I. p. 420.

[2] Devens. *Diss. de fungo cancroso ex verruca orto.*

7. **Verruca febrilis** [febrile warts], which erupts on the entire body with fever like an exanthem. See *variolas verrucosas.*

8. **Verruca cancrosa or maligna** [cancerous or malignant wart, skin cancer] is a wart that darkens or reddens, becoming painful and varicose, which turns into cancer.[2]

9. **Verrucae venereae** [venereal warts], looking similar to mulberries or raspberries, erupt on the face of venereals, as I have seen a number of times.

The successful treatment of verruca is obtained

1. by *ligature*, which can be carried out with the help of silk thread or horse bristle applied to the stalks of the wart;

2. by *excision*, with which verrucous cancer is cured;

3. by *caustics*, such as concentrated spirit of salt, spirit of nitre, caustic oil of camphor, with which the warts should be smeared by means of a small painter's brush twice a day;

4. by *burning*, a needle, heated by a candle, is fixed into the wart;

5. by *rubbing* the wart with black soap, with either milk or fig leaf, or with earwax;

6. by application of a *vesicatory plaster*, and tincture of cantharidin;

7. by *sympathetic remedies*. It is said that a wart disappears after being well rubbed with fruit, or meat, or blood dripping from the cut-off head of an eel and then burying those remedies in the ground. As far as I am concerned, this approach, having been tried fairly often, has not succeeded.

Clusters of warts often disappear of their own accord after the patient has been purged and is then given asafetida for several weeks. *Venereal* warts are treated as venereal condylomata.

[1] Illustrious August Gottlieb Richter. *Surgery*. Book 1. p. 420.

[2] Caspar Maria von Devens. *Dissertation on cancerous fungus having arisen from a wart.*

Cornua Cutanea

Sunt excrescentiae callosae vel verrucosae, sed admodum magnae.

Subinde totum corpus vel pars corniculis exstantibus horret.[1]

Curantur spiritu nitri fumante, aut solutione argenti, qua cornua circa basim saepius illini debent, vel excisione cornuum e cute.

[1] *Ill.* Hallerus in suo magno opere physiologico observationes de cornibus cutaneis congessit. Tome v. p. 30. Ex fronte cornu natum refert Zacut. ex maxilla Bartholin, ex capite duo cornua Leigh. cornu 9 unciarum de capite feminae desectum Thoresbi, undique ex cute capitis Ingrassias, ex omnibus digitis, *Phil. Trans.*, ex femore vetulae *Journal. de Medic. & Histoire de la Chirurgie*, ex vulnere genu, Benedictus, undique ex manibus, pedibus, capite & fronte, Ingrassias, ex articulis artuum, natibus & mammis Sylvius.

~~~~~~~~~~

Hystriciasis

Est papillarum, setis rigidis, ut hystrix habet, similium, copiosa progenies in cute.[1]

Nec *causa* nec *curatio* miri hujus morbi cutanei nota est.

[1] In Anglia fuit homo visus, cujus caput setis rigidis, pellucidis, 6 lineas longis, 2 vel 3 crassis, horrescebat. Hae setae quovis autumno decidebant. Is genuit 5 filios eodem morbo affectos. V. *Phil. Trans*, n. 424, & *Journal. de Med.* Mars 1756.

~~~~~~~~~~

Cornua Cutanea [cutaneous horn]

Cornua cutanea are callused or verrucous growths, but quite large.

Sometimes, the entire body or part of it looks bristly with projecting little horns.[1]

They are treated with steaming spirit of nitre; or with a solution of silver with which the horns should be smeared around the base fairly often; or by cutting off the horns from the skin.

[1] The Illustrious Haller in his great physiological work collected observations on cutaneous horns. Book V, page 30. Abraham Zacutus reports a horn produced spontaneously from the forehead; Bartholin reports the same from the maxilla; Leigh reports two horns from the head; Thoresby reports a horn of nine ounces cut from a woman's head; Ingrassias reports corns from all sides of the skin of the head; there is a report in *Philosophical Transactions* stating that horns grew from all digits; a report in the *Journal of Medicine and the History of Surgery* of a horn growing from the femur of an old woman; Benedict reports a horn growing from a wound of the knee; Ingrassius reports the same from everywhere on the hands, feet, head, and forehead, and Sylvius reports the same from joints of limbs, buttocks, and the breasts.

~~~~~~~~~~

Hystriciasis [ichthyosis hystrix]

Hystriciasis is an abundance of papules with rigid bristles, similar to what a porcupine has that multiplies all over the skin.[1]

Neither the cause nor the cure of this astonishing skin disease is known.

[1] In England there was a man seen whose head was bristled over with rigid, translucent hairs, 6 lines long (1/2 inch), 2 or 3 lines thick (1/6 to 1/4 inch). These bristles fell out every autumn. He sired 5 children affected by the same disease. See *Philosophical Transactions*, number 424, and *Journal of Medicine*, March 1756.

~~~~~~~~~~

Condylomata

Sunt verrucae molles, quae circa anum & pudenda utriusque sexus excrescunt.

Respectu originis, figurae, magnitudinis & indolis admodum variae sunt hae excrescentiae.

Species esse solent:

1. **Condylomata venerea**, quae vix dolent & ex praegressis vel praesentibus aliis symptomatibus, venereis noscuntur.

2. **Condylomata haemorrhoidalia**, quae absentia symptomatum venereorum, atque praegressis haemorrhoidibus noscuntur.

3. **Condylomata maligna**. Haec dolent, livent, & in cancrum abeunt; ex male tractatis condylomatibus aliis nascuntur.

Respectu *figurae* vocantur condylomata.

1. *Ficus* vel *sycocis*, quae magna sunt & ficus figuram referunt.
2. *Cristae*, quae cristis gallinaceis similia sunt.
3. *Tymus*, quae flores tymi vel brassicam caulifloram repraesentant.

Causa proxima, est evolutio vasorum, quae papillas cutaneas constituunt.

Curatio. Condylomata *venerea* praeter internum mercurii usum quotidie bis solutione saturata mercurii sublimati, vel aqua caustica ad condylomata ope penicilli illini & illico linimento mercuriali obtegi debent. Condylomata autem jam nimis *magna* & *sarcotica*, cultro, forfice vel si petiolata sunt, ligatura aufferuntur [*sic*].

Condylomata *haemorrhoidalia* linimento catheretico, ex pulvere aluminis usti, opii, flammulae jovis cum unguento de linaria subactis, saepe curantur.

Condylomata [genital warts]

Condyloma are soft warts that grow around the anus and groin of both sexes.

With respect to origin, shape, size, and quality, there are a great many varieties of these growths.

The customary species are:

1. **Condyloma venerea** [venereal condyloma], which are barely painful and recognized as being preceded by or presenting along with other venereal symptoms.

2. **Condyloma haemorrhoidalia** [hemorrhoidal condyloma], which are recognized by the absence of venereal symptoms and having been preceded by hemorrhoids.

3. **Condyloma maligna** [malignant condyloma]. These are painful, bluish, and evolve into cancer; other condyloma often arise from the ones treated for this malady.

Condyloma are named with respect to their shape:

1. *ficus* or *sycosis*, which are large and bring to mind the shape of a fig.

2. *cristas*, which are similar to the crest of a fowl.

3. *tymus*, which resemble the flowers of thyme or cauliflower.

The proximate cause is from the unfolding of the vessels, which make up the cutaneous papules.

Treatment. Besides the internal use of mercury twice daily, *venereal* condyloma should be smeared with a saturated solution of sublimate mercury or caustic water, applied to the condyloma with the help of a painter's brush and immediately covered with a mercury liniment. However, condyloma that are already too *large* and fleshy are removed with a knife, scissors, or, if there are stalks, by ligature.

Hemorrhoidal condyloma are often treated with a corrosive liniment made from burned alum dust, opium, and flammula jovis, with an ointment from cultivated linaria.

Condyloma *malignum* ut cancer tractetur.

Condylomata *indurata* cepa oleo cocta emolliantur, ac dein pulvere fabinae conspergantur.[1]

[1] *Neue Versuche und Bemerkungen einer Gesellschaft zu Edimburg.* 3. B. p. 373.

~~~~~~~~~~

Frambaesia

Est morbus, in quo praegressis pustulis variolis valde si milibus excrescentiae fungosae, mori fructus referentes, praecipue in plantis pedum quandoque in toto fere corpore excrescunt.[1]

Morbus hicce americanis est endemius & licet mercurio curetur & per coitum inficiat, tamen venereus non censetur, nam quos semel exercuit, si bene ab eo curati sint, hos non amplius aggreditur; genitalia maxime afficit. Morbo inveterato sese adjungunt ulcera dysepulota, exostoses, caries, anchyloses & macies.

Curatio. A morbi initio usque ad finem decocta purificantia ex herbis saponaceis & leniter sudorifera medicamenta dentur. Post integrum fungorum incrementum, quod intra 3 menses ordinarie contingit, solutio sublimati corrosivi cum decocto saturatissimo sarsaparillae detur. Sanato toto morbo *princeps fungus*, qui *Mamapian* Guineensibus dicitur, solutione caustica consumi debet. Nigritae fuliginem lebetum aeneorum, succo limoniorum dilutam, ulceribus & fungis applicant.

[1] Americani has excrescentias Pians seu fungos dicunt hinc Cel. Cartheuserus hunc morbum *lepram fungiferam* nominat. Cel. Schilling de morbo in Europa pene ignoto, quem *Americani vocant Iaws. 1770. Trajecti ad rhenum & Cel. Nielen, von den indianischen Pocken, oder den Sogenannten Jaws. Vide Sammlung fur praktische Aerzte. 7 Band 2 und 3 Stück.*
~~~~~~~~~~

Malignant condyloma may be managed as cancer.

Indurated condyloma should be softened with boiled onion oil, and then sprinkled with savin powder.[1]

[1] *New experiments and observations of a society in Edinburgh.* Book III, p. 373.

~~~~~~~~~~

Frambaesia [yaws]

Frambaesia is a disease in which variola pustules vigorously progress into innumerable spongy growths, bringing to mind the fruit of the mulberry, especially on the soles of the feet, and sometimes they grow out over very nearly the entire body.[1]

This disease is endemic to Americans. Although it may be cured with mercury and may infect through coitus, and it mostly affects the genitals, nevertheless, it is not reckoned to be venereal because those whom it has plagued once—if they are able to be totally cured from it—are not attacked again. In this chronic disease, associated features include scarring ulcers, exostoses, caries, stiff joints, and wasting.

Treatment. From the beginning to the end of the disease, purifying decoctions made from soapy herbs and mild sweat-promoting medications may be given. After the complete growth of the fungus, which normally occurs within three months, a solution of corrosive sublimate should be given with a very saturated decoction of sarsaparilla. After the whole disease has been cured, *the primary lesion*, which is called by the Guineans *Mamapian*, should be destroyed with a caustic solution. The Nigritae apply the soot of bronze cauldrons, diluted with juice of limoniums, to the ulcers and fungi.

[1] Americans call these excrescences *pians* or fungi, hence the celebrated Cartheuserus names this disease fungus-bearing leprosy. The celebrated Schilling wrote in 1770 about a disease almost unknown in Europe which the Americans call yaws. After yaws was transported across the Rhine, the celebrated Nielen wrote about the Indian smallpox or the so-called yaws. See *Collection for Practicing Physicians* Volume 7. Part 2 and 3.
~~~~~~~~~~

CLASSIS X. ULCERA CUTANEA

Sunt superficialia ulcera seu solutiones continui purulentae in sola externa cutis superficie.

Genera hujus classis sunt.

Excoriatio Purulenta

Est ulcus superficiale & purulentum in cutis superficie. Species sunt:

1. **Excoriatio bullosa**. Ea est, quae cum bulla, vi aut sua sponte rupta, incipit. Exigit linimentum molle.

2. **Excoriatio a vesicatorio**. V. *Bulla a vesicatorio.*

3. **Excoriatio acrimoniosa**. Materia venerea, cancrosa, scabiosa vel alia cuti illita praevia inflammatione ulcus superficiale excitat.

Curatio exigit unguentum molle cum specifico contra detectam acrimoniam.

4. **Excoriatio papillarum in mammis**, quae a violenta suctione infantis aut acrimonia ejus salivae oritur.

Curatur butyro cacao vel pulvere insperso ex amylo, bolo armena & saccharo albo.

~~~~~~~~~~

Intertrigo

Est excoriatio genitalium vel alius partis, madens, & rubens, ab urinae vel sudoris acrimonia.
~~~~~~~~~~

CLASS X. CUTANEOUS ULCERS

Cutaneous ulcers are superficial ulcers or the dissolution from continuous purulence on the external surface of the skin only.

The *genera* of this class are:

Excoriatio Purulenta [purulent erosion]

Excoriatio purulenta is a superficial and purulent ulcer on the surface of the skin. The species are:

1. **Excoriatio bullosa** [excoriated blister]. This begins with a blister that ruptures spontaneously or with force. It requires a soft liniment.

2. **Excoriatio a vesicatorio** [excoriation by vesicatorio]. See *Bulla from vesicatory.*

3. **Excoriatio acrimoniosa** [acrimonious excoriation]. Venereal, cancerous, scabious or other substances, having been smeared on the skin unintentionally, cause a superficial ulcer in areas of preceding inflammation.

The treatment requires a gentle unguent specifically for the detected acrimony.

4. **Excoriatio papillarum in mammis** [excoriation of the nipple], which arise from vehement suction by the infant or the acrimony of its saliva.

It is treated with cocoa butter or sprinkled with powder made from starch, Armenian bole, and white sugar.

~~~~~~~~~~

Intertrigo

Intertrigo is an excoriation of the genitals or of another part, dripping and reddening, from acrimony of urine or sweat.
~~~~~~~~~~

Species sunt:

1. **Intertrigo genitalium** est lactentibus familiaris, oritur custodum negligentia, quae infantes in linteis, urina faecibusque conspurcatis, diu sine purgatione relinquunt.

Curatio exigit diligentem mutationem linteorum mundorum, & inspersionem pulveris amyli, lycopodii, vel boli armenae.

2. **Intertrigo scroti** sudantibus a sudore acri, & in incontinentia urinae adultis etiam familiaris est.
3. **Intertrigo subaxillaris.** Tempore aestivo a sudore acri cavum subaxillare saepe excoriatur.
4. **Intertrigo auricularis**. Infantes retro aures saepe excoriari solent, praesertim si scabie capitis laborant.

Curatio intertriginis exigit, ut excretio non subito impediatur, sed prius datis purgantibus locus excoriatus ab initio cerato vel butyro cacao, in fluxu servetur dein bolo armena inspergatur. Cerussa plumbi evitetur.

~~~~~~~~~~

Aphthae

Sunt parva, albicantia & superficialia ulcuscula in oris cavo, vel, quod rarius est, in genitalibus, primis viis, aut trachea.

Incipiunt aphthae sub forma vesicularum miliarium albarum, quae in apice foraminulum gerunt, dein collabuntur & aliquantum latescunt.

Species aphtharum sunt diversae respectu *loci* & *indolis.*

1. **Aphthae infantiles**. Lactentibus sunt familiares & a lacte corrupto infantis vel nutricis fieri creduntur. Palatum, linguam & genas internas obsident, non raro simul in genitalibus observantur.
~~~~~~~~~~

The species are:

1. **Intertrigo genitalium** [intertrigo of the genitals, diaper dermatitis] is familiar to lactating women as it arises from negligence by the caregivers who leave the infants in diapers befouled with urine and feces for a long time without cleansing.

The treatment requires diligent changing of clean linens and sprinkling of starch powder, lycopodia, or Armenian bole.

2. **Intertrigo scroti** [scrotal intertrigo] is familiar even to adults sweating an acrid sweat and with urinary incontinence.

3. **Intertrigo subaxillaris** [underarm intertrigo]. The vault of the underarm is often excoriated from an acrid sweat in the summertime.

4. **Intertrigo auricularis** [auricular intertrigo]. Infants are often in the habit of scratching behind the ears, especially if suffering from scabies of the head.

The treatment of intertrigo requires that excretion not be hindered suddenly, but, after the purgatives have been given, first the excoriated place should be continuously coated, smeared from the beginning with cerate or cocoa butter, and then sprinkled with Armenian bole. White lead is to be avoided.

~~~~~~~~~~

Aphthae [aphthous ulcers]

Aphthae are small, whitish, and superficial ulcers in the oral cavity, or more rarely in the genitals, primis viis, or trachea.

The aphthae begin in the form of small white miliary vesicles which develop a small opening at the apex, then collapse and widen somewhat.

The species of aphthae are diverse with respect to location and quality:

1. **Aphthae infantiles** [infantile aphthae] are familiar to unweaned infants, and they are believed to be caused by corrupt milk of the wet nurse given to the infant. They besiege the palate, tongue, and buccal mucosa, and not rarely are they observed on the genitals at the same time.
~~~~~~~~~~

Infantes lac sugere recusant, pervigiles & febrientes saepe fiunt, nutrices calorem oris infantis sub lactatione sentiunt, & non raro papillae mammarum aphthis inficiuntur.

Curatio exigit, ut infans syrupo de spina cervina vel manato purgetur, & ut os aphthosum aqua vitriolata cum melle rosacco [*sic*] vel solutione boracis, quae etiam interne dari potest, saepius de die eluatur.

Nutrix simul purgetur & bibat decoctum bardanae atque ab omnibus acidis, acribus & vino abstineat.

2. **Aphthae adultorum**. In palato, interna superficie genarum vel labiorum, subinde in tonsillis vel faucium cavo una vel plures *magnae* aphthae oriuntur. Apex & latera linguae punctis hinc inde pertusa videntur. Locus aphthae sub masticatione aut deglutitione acriter dolet. Febris abest.[1]

Curatio est ut in aphthis infantum.

3. **Aphthae febriles**. Erumpunt cum febre acuta & non solum oris cavum, sed subinde simul fauces, tracheam, aesophagum, atque primas vias obsident. V. apud Authores descriptionem *febris aphthosae.*

4. **Aphthae gangraenosae**, livent & faetent: observantur in angina gangraenosa, & febre maligna. Exigunt collutorium ex cortice peruviano, ruta & camphora.

5. **Aphthae venereae** ulcera superficialia, muco gryseo tecta, faciunt: noscuntur signis luis venereae, curantur collutorio ex amylo & mercurio gummoso, & decocto sarsaparillae.

6. **Aphthae mercuriales**, quae cum ptyalismo & oris foetore erumpunt, praesertim orificia ductuum salivalium *Stenoni* afficiunt.

Curantur purgantibus, balneis calidis, & decocto emolliente lacteo.

Infants refuse to suckle milk, often becoming restless and feverish; the wet nurses sense a warmth in the mouth of the infant while breastfeeding, and not rarely suffer from aphthae of the mammary papillae.

Treatment requires that the infant be purged with syrup of spina cervina or by hand, and that the aphthous mouth be rinsed often throughout the day with vitriol water with rose-honey or a solution of borax, which can also be given internally.

The nurse should at the same time be purged and drink a decoction of burdock root and abstain from all acids, harsh foods, and wine.

2. **Aphthae adultorum** [adult aphthae]. On the palate, the superficial interior of the cheeks or lips, from time to time on the tonsils or the vault of the throat, one or more *large* ulcers arise. The apex and sides of the tongue appear perforated with dots at random. The site of the aphthae is sharply painful with chewing or swallowing. Fever is absent.[1]

The treatment is the same as for apththae infantum.

3. **Aphthae febriles** [febrile aphthae] erupt with acute fever, not only in the oral cavity, but sometimes they simultaneously besiege the throat, trachea, and esophagus, as well as the gastrointestinal tract. See the writings of authors who have described *aphthous fever.*

4. **Aphthae gangraenosae** [gangrenous aphthae] become livid and smell bad; they are observed in angina gangrenosa and malignant fever. They require a collutorium made of Peruvian bark, rue, and camphor.

5. **Aphthae venereae** [venereal aphthae] make a superficial ulcer covered with a gray mucous; they are known as a sign of syphilis; they are treated with a collutorium from starch, mercurius gummosus, and boiled sarsaparilla.

6. **Aphthae mercuriales** [mercurial aphthae] erupt with ptyalism and bad breath, primarily affecting the orifices of Stensen's salivary ducts.

They are treated with purgatives and warm baths and softened with boiled milk.

7. **Aphthae scorbuticae** noscuntur stomacace gingivarum & aliis scorbuti signis.

Curantur interne antiscorbuticis, externe melle rosaceao, & spiritu salis tangantur, atque dein tinctura gingivali eluantur.

Huc pertinet *cancer aquaticus*, qui magna est aphtha, cito in gangraenam buccarum vel labiorum transiens, curatur etiam interno & externo usu spiritus salis marini.

8. **Aphthae symptomaticae** sunt illae, quae febri miliari, petechiali, dysenteriae, phthysi, gangraenae pulmonis & cancro superveniunt, atque utplurimum incurabiles sunt.

[1] Vidi nuper in quodam pago multos rusticos os admodum habuisse aphthosum, cum lac, e vaccis aphthosis mulsum, frigidum tempore messis potarent, nobiliores autem hujus pagi, qui lac bibebant calefactum, aphthis non afficiebantur.

Fissurae

Sunt solutiones lineares, siccae vel humidae, in cuticula vel cute. Species sunt:

1. **Fissurae a frigore**, quae in labiis oris, manibus, pedibusque hieme observantur.

Curantur unguento ad perniones.

2. **Fissurae labiorum a vento**, quae tempore ventoso itinerantibus contingunt.

Curantur butyro cacao vel unguento ad labia.

3. **Fissurae ab acribus**. Ut accidunt ancillis lixivium calidum incaute tractantibus. Curantur butyro. Fissurae, quae in manibus ab *atramento typographico* oriebantur, unguento alcalino curabantur.

7. **Aphthae scorbuticae** [scorbutic aphthae] are recognized by inflammation of the gums and other signs of scurvy.

They are treated internally with antiscorbutics; externally they should be smeared with rose-honey and spirit of salt, and then rinsed with gingival tincture.

Cancer aquaticus belongs here, which is a large aphthous ulcer that quickly transforms into gangrene of the inner cheeks or lips; it is also treated by the internal and external use of the spirit of sea salt.

8. **Aphthae symptomaticae** [symptomatic aphthae] are those aphthae that accompany miliary fever, petechiae, dysentery, phthisis, pulmonary gangrene, and cancer. They are nearly impossible to cure.

[1] I recently saw in a certain province many rustics who kept a very ulcerated mouth when they drank milk, drawn from ulcerated cows, which was cold at harvest time; however, the nobles of this province who were drinking warm milk were not affected by the aphthous ulcers.

~~~~~~~~~~

Fissurae [fissures]

Fissurae are dry or wet linear erosions on the cuticle or skin. The species are:

1. **Fissurae a frigore** [fissures from the cold] are observed on the lips, the hands, and the feet in the winter.

They are treated with the unguent for pernio (chilblains).

2. **Fissurae labiorum a vento** [fissures of the lip from the wind] befall travelers in the windy season.

They are treated with cocoa butter or unguent for lips.

3. **Fissurae ab acribus** [fissures from irritants] happens to maidservants incautiously handling warm lye. It is treated with butter. Fissures that arose on the hands from *printer's ink* were treated with alkaline unguent.
~~~~~~~~~~

4. **Fissurae papillarum mammae**. Nutricibus a violenta & perpetua suctione infantis sunt familiares.

Curatio exigit abstinentiam aliqualem a lactatione, butyrum cacao & pulverem ad mammillas, qui ex amylo, sacharo [*sic*] & bolo armena constat.

~~~~~~~~~~

Rhagades

Sunt malignae, siccae & profundae fissurae cutaneae.

Species sunt:

1. **Rhagades venereae**, quae in volis manuum plantisque pedum, atque circa ani & vulvae orificium oriri solent. Noscuntur morbis venereis praegressis.

Curantur admodum difficulter. Interne dentur mercurialia. Externe pomatum ex mercurio praecipitato rubro vel albo, aqua phagaedenica vel solutio saturata mercurialis adhibeatur.

2. **Rhagades leprosae** sunt, quae in lepra, elephantiasi & frambaesia totam fere cutem occupant.

3. **Rhagades anonimae**, quas in hominibus nec venereis, nec leprosis ex causa adhuc incognita in volis manuum vidi. Cuticula crassa, rhagadibus plena erat, gluten copiosum ex rhagidibus exsudabat. Nec mercurius, nec alia medicamenta profuere.

A decocto saturato chaerophilli interne & externe adhibito saepius cuticula cum rhagadibus quandoque secessit, laudatur etiam auripigmentum, cum unguento digestivo.

Nuper haec curatio tentata fuit:[1]

1. Lavetur manus *lixivio cinerum* ex ligno.

2. Dein *aqua pulviali [sic] destillata* abluantur.
~~~~~~~~~~

4. **Fissurae papillarum mammae** [fissures of the nipples] are familiar to wet nurses from vehement and constant sucking by the infant.

Treatment requires abstinence from any kind of lactation, and for the breasts; cocoa butter and powder consisting of starch, sugar, and Armenian bole.

~~~~~~~~~~

Rhagades

Rhagades are destructive, dry, and deep cutaneous fissures.

The species are:

1. **Rhagades venereae** [venereal rhagades], usually arise on the palms or soles of the feet and also around the orifice of the anus and vulva. They are recognized in advanced venereal diseases.

It is very difficult to treat. Internally, mercurials should be given. Externally, an ointment of red or white precipitated mercury, phagedenic water, or a saturated solution of mercurials.

2. **Rhagades leprosae** [leprous rhagades] are those rhagades that spread over almost the entire skin in lepra, elephantiasis, and frambesia.

3. **Rhagades anonimae** [rhagades without name] which I saw on the palms from an as-yet-unknown cause in men with neither venereal disease nor leprosy. With the cuticle thickened, it was full of rhagades, with an abundance of viscous substance exuding from the rhagades. Neither mercury nor other medicines were beneficial.[1]

By means of a saturated decoction of chaerophyllum employed fairly often internally and externally, the cuticle with rhagades has sometimes separated; orpiment is also recommended, with dissolving ointment.

Recently, this treatment has been attempted:

1. Let the hands be washed with *lye from wood ashes.*

2. Next, they should be cleansed with *distilled rainwater.*
~~~~~~~~~~

3. Dein manus sequenti unguento illinantur. Rx. Sevi vervecini, cerae albae, succi pomorum borsdorfensium & olei olivarium p. aequales, in unguentum redigantur, hocce chirothecae illinantur, quibus manus die noctuque induantur.

4. Interne *Tinctura antimonii Thediana* & ad vesperas *gummi guajaci* cum gr. v. *saponis antimonialis* detur.

4. **Rhagades seniles**, quae in senibus a cutis siccitate & transpiratione suppressa oriuntur.

Curatio prior tentetur.

[1] Cel. Theden. *Bemerkungen.* 2. *Theil.* p. 262. Rhagades digitorum & volae manus jam a 10 annis vexantes in proprio corpore hac methodo sanavit.

3. Then the hands should be smeared with the following ointment: Rx. Equal parts of tallow of castrated ram, white wax, juice of the bors-dorf apple, and olive oil, reduced into an ointment; the hands should be covered day and night with gloves in which this ointment has been smeared.

4. Internally, *Theden's tincture of antimony,* and in the evenings *guaiac gum* with five grams of *antimonial soap* is given.

4. **Rhagades seniles** [senile rhagades], which arises in the elderly from dried skin and suppressed transpiration.

The previous treatment should be tried.

[1] The celebrated Theden. *New Remarks and Experience of Wound Medicine and Medicinal Science.* Erster-Dritter Theil. part 2, page 262. He cured with this method rhagades of the fingers and palms of the hands of his own body that had been vexing him for ten years.

CLASSIS XI. VULNERA CUTANEA

Sunt vulnera, quae solam cutem laedunt.

Huc maxime pertinent.

Excoriatio Cruenta

Est cuticulae vel cutis a partibus subjacentibus cruenta & violenta separatio.

Species excoriationis cruentae sunt:

1. **Excoriatio a violento attritu**, quae supra partes ossibus sustentatas, ut supra spinas tibiarum, cranium aut digitorum articulos frequentissime contingit. Haec excoriatio summe dolorifica est, & paulo post multum inflammatur.

Nihil utilius est quam fomentum ex aqua Thediana vel ex vino tepido cum aliquot guttis extracti saturni. Ipsa viva excoriatio parva portione emplastri anglicani tegatur. Evitentur spiritus & unguenta praesertim in corporibus cachecticis, in his ab excoriatione violenta saepe magnum ulcus erysipelatosum excitatur.

Huc etiam pertinent *Excoriatio* volae *manus* a labore, aut *pedis* plantae ab itinere, excoriatio in interna & summa *femorum* parte ab equitatione, & in regione *ossis sacri* aut calce pedis a longo & duro decubitu. V. *Erythema ab attritu.*

2. **Excoriatio unguicularis**, quae ab unguibus hominis, fellis, vel alius animalis infligitur. Longam & cruentam repraesentat lineam, sic etiam infantes, quibus cutis in capite vel alio loco moleste prurit, unguibus locum prurientem adeo fricare solent, ut sanguis ex cute erumpat.

~~~~~~~~~~
~~~~~~~~~~

CLASS XI. CUTANEOUS WOUNDS

Cutaneous wounds are wounds that only damage the skin.

The main ones that belong here are:

Excoriatio Cruenta [bloody excoriation]

Excoriatio cruenta is a bloody and violent separation of the cuticle or skin from its underlying parts.

The species of *excoriatio cruenta* are:

1. **Excoriatio a violento attritu** [excoriation from violent injury, laceration], which occurs most frequently above the parts supported by bones, such as over the spines of the tibias, the cranium, or joints of the fingers or toes. This laceration is extremely pain producing and, after a short time, much inflamed.

Nothing is more useful than a poultice of Thedian water or tepid wine with some drops of lead extract. Let the living excoriation itself be covered with a small portion of English plaster. Spirits and ointments should be avoided, especially in cachectic bodies, since in them large erysipelatous ulceration is often caused by violent excoriation.

Here also belongs *excoriation* of the *palm* from labor, or on the *sole* from travel, or excoriation on the inner and highest part of the *femurs* from horseback riding, and in the *sacral area* or heel from a long and difficult bed rest. See *Erythema ab attritu.*

2. **Excoriatio unguicularis** [excoriation from nails, scratch], which is inflicted by the nails of man, cats, or other animals. It is characterized by a long and bloody line; thus, even infants, whose skin of the scalp or other places itch intensely, customarily scratch the itchy place with nails to such a degree that blood might erupt from the skin.

~~~~~~~~~~
~~~~~~~~~~

Scissura

Est solutio cutis, cruentam lineam referens, acuto instrumento inflicta.

Curatur optime, si vulnus emplastro anglicano uniatur.

~~~~~~~~~~

Pressura

Est cutis intra ungues digitorum compressio.

Partes nerveae sic pressae ut labia, facies, aut mammae non raro tuberculum durum inflammatum retinent, quod in cancrum degenerare potest.

Curatio exigit, ut illico vino tepido inflammatio resolvatur.

Morsus

Est cutis intra dentes animalis solutio cruenta.

Morsus Species sunt, *morsus simplex* & *morsus ab animali rabioso* vel *irrato.* Eadem mala producit ac pressura cum unguibus. Sed morsus animalis *irrati* vel *rabiosi* praeterea rabiem inducit. V. *Vulnera venenata*, quae in *chirurgia* descripsi.

Curatio morsus simplicis exigit balsamum Arcaei.

~~~~~~~~~~

Punctura

Est solutio cutis per acum, aliudve instrumentum acutum. Species sunt:

1. **Punctura simplex**. Si cutis per acum pungitur, una alterave guttula sanguinis exit, quae aëre exsiccatur & vulnus intra diem sua sponte, si sanguine tectum manet, sanatur.

Scissura [laceration]

Scissura is a split in the skin, resembling a bloody line, inflicted by a sharp instrument.

It is optimally treated if the wound is joined together with English plaster.

~~~~~~~~~~

Pressura [pinched skin]

Pressura is the pinching of the skin between the fingertips.

Highly sensitive areas—the lips, face, or breasts—pressed in such a way often hold in place a firm inflamed nodule which can degenerate into cancer.

Treatment requires that the inflammation be resolved with warm wine on that very spot.

Morsus [bite]

Morsus is a bloody tear in the skin by the tooth of animals.

The species of bites are a *simple bite* and a *bite from a rabid* or *angry animal.* It produces the same injury as pinching with fingertips. But the bite of an *angry* or *rabid* animal in addition causes rabies. See the *poisonous wounds* which I have described in my surgical writings.

The treatment of a simple bite requires balsam of Arcaeus.

~~~~~~~~~~

Punctura [puncture wound]

Punctura is an injury to the skin by a needle or other sharp instrument. The species are:

1. **Punctura simplex** [simple puncture wound]. If the skin is punctured by a needle, one or two little drops of blood come out, which is dried by the air and the wound is healed spontaneously within a day, if it remains covered with blood.

2. **Punctura complicata cum cuspide fracta et intra vulnus relicta**, ut saepe cum festucis ligneis contingit.

Curatio exigit, ut corpus heterogeneum e vulnere extrahatur. Si haec extractio impossibilis est, vulnus lanceola dilatetur, aut excitetur vulneris suppuratio, sic festuca fere sua sponte exit.

3. **Punctura a vipera venenata vel non venenata**. Noscitur duabus puncturis juxta se locatis. Viperae venenatae fere omnes duos in ore gerunt aculeos, plicatiles & cavos, quorum basis premit folliculos duos, succo venenato turgidos, qui in vulnus effunditur, dum animal mordet.

Puncturae viperarum non venenatarum leves & sine periculo sunt, venenatarum autem puncturae pessima symptomata & saepe brevi mortem inferunt. V. *Toxicologiam.*

4. **Punctura ab hirudine**. Vulnus ab hoc verme illatum est triangulare, subin etiam ablato hirudine diu sanguinem plorat.

Curatur suasponte [*sic*] vel applicato vino calido.

~~~~~~~~~~

Ictus ab Insecto

Est punctura ab insecto illata.

Species sunt:

1. **Ictus a pediculo** facit parvum stigma cutaneum, cujus peripheria albescit.

2. **Ictus a pulice** stigma facit, cujus ambitus late rubet. An pediculus solum sanguinem, & pulex solum serum ex inflicto vulnere exsugit?
~~~~~~~~~~

2. **Puncturum complicata cum cuspide fracta et intra vulnus relicta** [complicated puncture wound with broken point retained in the wound], as often happens with wooden sticks.

Treatment requires that the heterogeneous body be extracted from the wound. If this extraction is impossible, the wound may be widened with a small lance, or suppuration of the wound may result, so that the splinter exits the wound almost on its own.

3. **Punctura a vipera venenata vel non venenata** [puncture wound from a venomous or non-venomous snake]. It is recognized by two punctures located next to each other. Almost all venomous snakes have two folded and hollow fangs in the mouth, with the base of each pressing small sacs, swollen with poisonous juice, which pours out into the wound while the snake bites.

The punctures of non-venomous snakes are slight and without danger; however, the punctures of venomous snakes bring very bad symptoms and often a quick death. See *Toxicology*.

4. **Punctura ab hirudine** [puncture by leech]. The wound brought about by this worm is triangular; often, even after the leech has been removed, it weeps blood for a long time.

It is cured spontaneously or with an application of hot wine.

~~~~~~~~~~

Ictus ab Insecto [insect bite]

Ictus ab insecto is the puncture brought about by an insect.

The species are:

1. **Ictus a pediculo** [louse bite] makes a small cutaneous mark, whose periphery whitens.

2. **Ictus a pulice** [flea bite] makes a mark whose perimeter reddens extensively. Can it be that the louse sucks out only blood and the flea sucks out only serum from the inflicted wound?
~~~~~~~~~~

3. **Ictus a cimice, culice & vespa**, tubercula rubra & admodum prurientia relinquit in cute. Haec applicatione aquae frigidae, vel aceti curantur.

4. **Ictus a scorpione**. Hic multis animalibus lethalis est, sed hominibus raro, nisi magnus nervus pungatur. Laudatur externe oleum scorpionum, quod autem non semper symptomata aufert.

5. **Ictus a tarantula**. Hujus ictus dolorem, dein tumorem livescentem, paucos post dies crusta nigricante obsitum, excitat; accedunt somnolentia, oppressionis anxietatisque sensus, & demum dolores in singulis corporis articulis, sed nunquam effrenis saltandi cupiditas homines demorsos incessit, ut vulgo narratur. Haec symptomata diaphoreticis curantur.

6. **Ictus a furia infernali**. Hoc insectum est vermiforme tenuissimum & vix duas lineas longum. In Suecia ex aere delabitur, & momento citius tum in hominum, tum in jumentorum corpora penetrat, atque tam diros excitat dolores, ut miseri homines quandoque intra horae quadrantem pereant, dantur tamen, qui diutius durant.

Cognoscitur locus ex stigmate, exiguo, fusco, & dolentissimo. Fenones lac recenter coagulatum partì vulneratae imponunt, sic dolor remittit, & insectum foras prorumpit: alii cultro locum incidunt, & animal extrahunt. V. *Toxicologiam.*

3. **Ictus a cimice, culice, and vespa** [bedbug, gnat, and wasp bites], leaves behind a red and extremely itchy nodule in the skin. These are treated with the application of cold water or vinegar.

4. **Ictus a scorpione** [scorpion bite]. This is lethal to many animals, but rarely to humans, unless a large nerve is punctured. Recommended for external use is the oil of scorpion, which, however, does not always take away the symptoms.

5. **Ictus a tarantula** [tarantula bite]. The bite of which causes pain, then a darkening knot, which after a few days is covered with a blackening crust; somnolence develops with a sense of oppression and anxiety, and eventually pain in every joint of the body, but never does the desire for frenetic dancing befall diseased men, as is commonly told. These symptoms are treated with diaphoretics.

6. **Ictus a furia infernali** [bite of the fury worm]. This insect is wormlike, very slender, and barely two lines long. In Sweden, it slips down from the air and then rather quickly penetrates the bodies of not only men but also beasts of burden. It causes such horrible pain that the wretched men perish sometimes within a quarter of an hour; it is conceded, however, that there are those who last longer.

The bite is recognized by a small, dark, and very painful mark. The country folk place freshly clotted milk on the wounded part; thus the pain remits, and the insect bursts forth out of the body; others cut the place with a knife and extract the animal. See *Toxicology*.

CLASSIS XII. INSECTA CUTANEA

Insecta & vermes, qui externam corporis superficiem infestare & in vel sub cute sedem figere solent, frequentissimi hi sunt:

1. **Pediculi capitis & pubis** in phtyriasi [*sic*].

2. **Acarus scabiei** in scabie verminosa.

3. **Acarus exulcerans** in scabie ferina.

4. **Larvae muscae leprae** in lepra nigritarum.

5. **Larvae muscae carnariae et vulgaris** in vulneribus, ulceribus, variolis & lepra.

6. **Pulex americanus** sub cute americanorum.

7. **Larvae aestrorum**, quae sub cute bovum & rhangiferorum tubera faciunt.

8. **Syrones** in pustulis manuum & pedum.

9. **Gordius medinensis** seu **dracunculus persarum**, qui in telam cellulosam penetrat.

10. **Lumbricus effractor**, qui quandoque ex abdomine effringit.

11. **Furia infernalis**, quae cutem perfodit ex aere delapsa.

12. **Ascarides**, quae intestinum rectum aut vulvam inhabitant.

13. **Scolopendra forficulata**, quae aures intrare amat.

14. **Hirudo**, qui cuti adhaerere solet hominum, qui stagna intrant.

~~~~~~~~~~
~~~~~~~~~~

CLASS XII. CUTANEOUS INSECTS

The insects and worms, which customarily infest the external surface of the body and fix a seat in or under the skin, are most frequently:

1. **Pediculi capitis et pubis** [lice of the head and of the pubic area] in phthiriasis.

2. **Acarus scabiei** [scabies mite] in verminous scabies.

3. **Acarus exulcerans** [ulcerating mite] in feral scabies.

4. **Larvae muscae leprae** [leprous maggots] in lepra of the Nigritae.

5. **Larvae muscae carnariae et vulgaris** [flesh-eating and common maggots] in wounds, ulcers, smallpox, and lepra.

6. **Pulex americanus** [human flea] under the skin of Americans.

7. **Larvae aestrorum** [botfly larva], which under the skin of cattle and caribou make a nodule.

8. **Sirones** in pustules of the hands and feet.

9. **Gordius medinensis** seu **dracunculus persarum** [Guinea worm or Persian dracunculus], which penetrates the cellular tissue.

10. **Lumbricus effractor**, which sometimes erupts from the abdomen.

11. **Furia infernalis**, which having descended from the air, perforates the skin.

12. **Ascarides**, which inhabit the rectum or vulva.

13. **Scolopendra forficulata**, which tends to enter the ear.

14. **Hirudo**, which customarily sticks to the skin of men who enter stagnant water.

~~~~~~~~~~
~~~~~~~~~~

Phthiriasis

Est morbus, in quo cutis vel aliae partes ingenti pediculorum copia obsidentur.

Haec insecta cutem puncturis, pruritu, sordibus, ulcusculisque valde discruciant.

Species sunt:

1. **Phthiriasis capitis**. Est infantibus familiaris, cum scabie, & porrigine furfuracea capitis conjunctus morbus. Capilli utplurimum *lendibus* copiosissimis, quae *ovula* pediculorum sunt, obsidentur.

Curatio exigit frequentem pectinationem & purificationem capitis, atque inspersionem seminis petroselini, sabadillae.

2. **Phthiriasis pubis**. In pilis pubis, scroti & inguinum pediculi lati, quos *platulas* seu *morpiones* appellant, observantur. Hi profunde cuti immerguntur, molestum pruritum excitant, at cutem non ut pediculi capitis exulcerant.

Curantur unguento neapolitano, aut solutione saturata mercuriali, vel pulvere seminis staphisagriae, vel infuso nicotianae.

3. **Phthiriasis superciliorum**. Pediculi, qui supercilia interdum inhabitant, sunt platulis similes.

Curantur aloe in aceto scillitico soluta, vel oleo spicae vel unguento mercuriali.

4. **Phthiriasis totius corporis**. Tota corporis superficies & omnia vestimenta, praesertim si lanea sunt, replentur pediculis & eorum lendibus.

Curatio exigit balnea ex nicotiana, inunctiones mercuriales cum oleo spicae, & nova vestimenta.

Interne cortex cum mercurio adhibeatur.

Phthiriasis [lice]

Phthiriasis is a disease in which the skin or other parts are inhabited by a huge multitude of lice.

These insects greatly torture the skin with punctures, itching, filth, and small ulcers.

The species are:

1. **Phthiriasis capitis** [head lice]. It is familiar to children with scabies and the concomitant malady of furfuraceous porrigo of the scalp. The scalp is nearly always teeming with nits, which are *eggs* of the lice.

The treatment requires frequent combing and cleansing of the head as well as sprinkling of the seeds of parsley and sabadilla.

2. **Phthiriasis pubis** [pubic lice]. They are broad-bodied lice, which are called *platulas* or *morpiones*, that are observed on the hairs of the pubis, scrotum, and inguinal areas. These are submerged deeply in the skin and cause an itchy irritation, but they do not ulcerate the skin as head lice do.

They are treated with Neapolitan ointment, or a saturated solution of mercurials, and either powdered seeds of Staphisagria or infused nicotianae.

3. **Phthiriasis superciliorum** [lice of eyebrow]. They are lice that occasionally inhabit the eyebrows and are similar to pubic lice.

They are treated with aloe dissolved in vinegar of squill and either oil of spike or mercurial ointment.

4. **Phthiriasis totius corporis** [lice of the entire body, body lice]. The entire surface of the body and all of the clothing, especially if woolen, are full of lice and their nits.

Treatment requires a bath with tobacco, anointings with mercury with oil of spike, and new clothing.

Internally, bark with mercury is used.

5. **Phthiriasis interna**. Est ea, in qua pediculi e diversis corporis locis exeunt, ut ex oculis, naribus, auribus, ore, cum urina, sputo, fecibus. Aegroti emaciantur & pereunt.

Curatio instituatur, ut in priori specie dixi.

Helmintiasis

Est morbus, in quo cutis, vel aliae partes externae ingenti vermium vel larvarum vermiformium copia obsidentur.

Species sunt:

1. **Helmintiasis cutanea**. Hic morbus endemius est Martinicanis, Westphalis, Transsylvanis & Acridophagis. Miseris hoc morbo affectis per magnam corporis partem vermiculi sub cute cuniculos agunt, & fere totius corporis pinguedinem consumunt, atque carnes hinc inde ad ossa usque devorant, adeo ut mors horrenda sequatur.

Curatio exigit interne & externe anthelmintica cum mercurialibus.

2. **Helmintiasis intestini recti, vulvae, urethrae, narium, aurium,** aut **gingivarum**.[1] Frequenti injectione tabaci, vel solutionis ex sale amaro & anthelminticis curatur.

3. **Helmintiasis ulcerum**. Vermes, qui in ulceribus, aut vulneribus sordidis, diu aeri expositis, negligenterque deligatis, potissimum aestate, rarissime autem hyeme reperiuntur, ovulis, a musca vulgari vel carnaria in ulcera depositis, originem debent. Hi vermiculi etiam in scabie humida, variolis maturis, atque in lepra inveniuntur.

Curatio exigit, ut ulcera bene eluantur, & mundentur, dein oleum terebinthinae, essentia aloes, vel elixirium vitrioli applicetur, vel mercurius dulcis inspergatur.

5. **Phthiriasis interna** [internal lice]. It is the species in which lice emerge from various parts of the body, such as the eyes, nares, ears, mouth, and with the urine, sputum, and feces. The infirm waste away and perish.

The treatment is administered as I have said for the lice of the whole body.

Helminthiasis

Helminthiasis is a disease in which the skin or other external parts are besieged by a large abundance of worms or worm larvae.

The species are:

1. **Helmintiasis cutanea** [cutaneous worms]. This disease is endemic among the people of Martinique, northern Germany, Transylvania, and among the locust-eaters. In the wretched men affected by this disease, the worms make tunnels under the skin through much of the body, and they consume the fat of nearly the whole body. They also devour the flesh in some places all the way down to the bones, to the point at which a horrendous death follows.

The treatment requires internally and externally an antihelmintics with mercurials.

2. **Helmintiasis intestini recti, vulvae, urethrae, narium, aurium,** aut **gingivarum**[1] [rectal, vulvar, urethral, nostril, ear, or gingival worms]. It is treated with frequent enema of tobacco or solution of bitter salt and antihelminthics.

3. **Helmintiasis ulcerum** [ulcer worms, myiasis]. These worms, which are in ulcers or dirty wounds exposed to the air for a long time and negligently bandaged, are found most commonly in the summer; very rarely, however, in the winter. They owe their origin to eggs deposited in the ulcer by the common fly or flesh fly. These small worms are also found in wet scabies, mature smallpox, and also in lepra.

The treatment requires that the ulcers be thoroughly washed and cleansed, then turpentine oil, aloe essence, or elixir of vitriol should be applied, or sweet mercury sprinkled on the ulcers.

[1] Vidi nuper infantem, cui gingivae ingenti copia vermium repletae erant, solutione salis amari banc [*sic*] helminthiasim intra paucos dies curavi.

~~~~~~~~~~

Malis

Tubera, quae insecta, vel vermes intra se recondunt, males dicuntur.

Species malium sunt:

1. **Malis pedicularis**, in capite & facie bulla visa fuit, quae incisa magnam copiam pediculorum continuit.

Curatio facta incisione exigit elutionem cum aqua vulneraria.

2. **Malis a pulice americano**. Hoc insectum in America degens vix conspicuum est, cutim peregrinantium maxime in cruribus subit, imo quandoque sub unguibus in cutem penetrat. Intra aliquot dies sub epidermide magnitudinem pisi acquirit & partem obsessam subinde ad ossa usque erodit.

Curatio exigit, ut insecta haec quotidie ope cultri acuti ex cute evellantur, & locus cinere tabaci combusti inspergatur. Ubi vero totum crus his insectis obsidetur, linteum oleo picis intinctum applicari debet, hoc remedio haec insecta cito separantur.

3. **Malis ab acaro sylvestri americano** etiam sic tractatur.

4. **Malis a gordio medinensi** seu **dracunculo persico**. Est vermis non solum circa Medinam & in Persia, sed in omnibus aestuosarum regionum lacubus obvius. In hominum cutem inter lavandum vel ambulandum in aqua lacustri se insinuare solet. Frequentissime crura & scrotum occupat.
~~~~~~~~~~

[1] I recently saw a baby whose gums were filled with an abundance of worms; I cured this case of helminthiasis with a solution of bitter salt within a few days.

~~~~~~~~~~

Malis

The swellings within which insects or worms conceal themselves are called *males* [plural of malis].

The species of *malis* are:

1. **Malis pedicularis** [swelling from lice], a bulla had been seen on the head and face, which, having been incised, was found to contain a great abundance of lice.

The treatment requires making an incision, then cleansing the wound with aqua vulneraria.

2. **Malis a pulice americano** [swelling from fleas]. This insect inhabiting America is scarcely conspicuous. It goes under the skin of travelers primarily on the legs, and other times it penetrates into the skin under the nails. Within a few days under the epidermis, it becomes the size of a pea and thereupon erodes the besieged part all the way down to the bones.

Treatment requires that these insects be plucked daily from the skin with the aid of a sharp knife, and the place sprinkled with the ash of burnt tobacco. But, when the whole leg is beset by these insects, a towel saturated with pitch oil should be applied, and by this remedy these insects are quickly removed.

3. **Malis ab acaro sylvestri americano** [swelling from the American forest mite] is also treated the same way.

4. **Malis a gordio medinensi** seu **dracunculo persico** [swelling from the dracunculus]. It is a worm encountered not only around Medina and in Persia, but also in all the lakes of the tropical regions. In human skin, it usually insinuates itself during bathing or wading in lake water. Most frequently, it attaches to the legs and scrotum.
~~~~~~~~~~

Hic vermis saepe ad plurium pedum longitudinem in tela cellulosa hominis, quem afficit, increscit, musculorum tractus sequi amat, subinde, quod pejus est, ossa serpentis adinstar amplectitur. Modo unus modo plures adesse deprehenduntur. Hic vermis per annum in corpore latitat, et praeter dolorem loci affecti nullum incommodum facit.

Non raro autem tumorem rubentem cum febre plurium dierum, quae nuncia est prodituri vermis, excitat. Exsurgit demum in tumore vesica pellucida, vel nigricans, ex qua rupta prosilit rostellum vermis, qui sensim magis erumpit, & ita extrahi paullatim potest.

Curatio exigit, ut tumor cataplasmate lacteo emolliatur, dein ut erumpentis vermis portio circa ligulam rotetur, sic intra 10 circiter dies totus vermis, cavendo ne rumpatur, extrahi potest. Ulcus extracto verme ut aliud curatur.

Enormis vermis longitudo, tarda maturatio, implicatio vermis circa ossa vel musculos, vermis ruptura, curationem longiorem, & difficiliorem reddunt.

5. **Malis a sironibus**. Hoc insectum intra cutim se insinuat & epidermidem in papulas attollit pruriginosas, rubras vel luteas, quae sensim exulcerantur. In planta pedis & vola manus sirones frequenter nidulari solent. Curatio exigit, ut sironus acu effodiantur, & dein locus sebo deligetur: alii solutionem salis amari, alii unguentum amarum cum mercurio dulci adhibent.

6. **Malis a lumbrico effractore**. Hic vermis ex intestinis in umbilico vel in inguinibus, praesertim in locis herniosis excitato abscessu erumpere solet. Relinquit fistulam subinde difficulter, subinde facile aqua thediana curabilem

~~~~~~~~~~
~~~~~~~~~~

This worm often increases to a length of several feet in the cellular layer of the person whom it affects; it tends to follow the tract of muscles, and sometimes—which is worse—it surrounds the bones in the fashion of a serpent. Sometimes only one, sometimes more are determined to be present. This worm lies hidden in the body for a year, and besides pain in the affected place, it causes no inconvenience.

However, not infrequently it causes a reddening tumor with fever for several days, which is a sign that a worm is about to be brought forth. Finally, a clear or blackening blister rises up into a swelling, from which, after being ruptured, the head of the worm springs forth. It breaks through rather slowly and thus can be extracted a little at a time.

The treatment requires that the swelling be softened with a milk plaster, then that the portion of the erupting worm be rotated by the throat; thus within about 10 days the entire worm, taking care it does not rupture, can be extracted. When the worm has been extracted, the ulcer is treated like any other.

Enormous worm length, slow maturation, worm entanglement around bones or muscles, and worm rupture render treatment that is rather long and difficult.

5. **Malis a sironibus** [swelling from the sirones]. This insect insinuates itself within the skin and raises the epidermis into red or yellow itchy pustules, which slowly ulcerate. In general, sirones frequently nest on the sole of the foot and palm of the hand. Treatment requires that the sironus be dug out with a needle and then the site be bound up with tallow; some people employ bitter salt solution, others bitter unguent with sweet mercury.

6. **Malis a lumbrico effractore** [swelling from *Lumbrico effractore*]. This worm usually erupts from the intestines into the navel or groin, particularly causing abscesses in the herniated places. It leaves behind a fistula, which is sometimes curable with difficulty; other times, it is easily curable with Thedian water.

~~~~~~~~~~
~~~~~~~~~~

Crinones

Sunt setae lineam longae, nigricantes & confertae, quae instar vermiculorum ex cute exprimi possunt.

Species sunt:

1. **Crinones infantum**. Cutis dorsi, brachiorum & crurum in infantibus athrophicis [*sic*] nigricantibus setis confertim obsidetur. Has setas aliqui pro vermiculis habent, & ideo *Comedones* vocant.

Curatio exigit, ut partes obsessae bile bubula vel manu ex calido oleo olivarum madida, vel aqua calida, cui parum farinae, aut pulveris cyprei additum est, alternis diebus fricentur.

2. **Crinones adultorum**. Puncta nigra referunt in facie, circa nasum, & in antica thoracis parte, quae puncta digitis ex cute pressa simulacra vermiculorum cum capite nigro exbibent. Sebum in foliculis cutaneis inspissatum & in externo apice corruptum, atque per porum excretorium glandulae expressum, hos vermiculos cum capite nigro repraesentat.

Curatur lotione saponacea ex sapone, vel oleo tartari per deliquium & expressione sebi, vel, quod optimum censetur, felle taurino.

Crinones

Crinones are a line of long, blackening, and clustered bristles that resemble small worms and can be expressed from the skin.

The species are:

1. **Crinones infantum** [infantile crinones, comedones]. The skin of the back, arms, and legs in atrophic infants is covered densely with blackening bristles. Some regard these bristles as worms and therefore call them comedones.

Treatment requires that the besieged areas be rubbed on alternating days with bovine bile either by a hand moistened with warm olive oil or with hot water to which an equal amount of flour or cyprus powder has been added.

2. **Crinones adultorum** [adult crinones, comedones]. These refer to black spots on the face, around the nose, and on the anterior part of the chest that present something similar to a small worm with a black head when expressed with the fingers from the skin. Sebum thickened in the follicles of the skin and corrupted at the outer tip, and squeezed through the excretory pore of the gland brings to mind these worms with a black head.

It is treated by a foamy washing with soap or with oleo tartari per deliquium and the expression of sebum, or, what is considered to be the best, ox gall.

CLASSIS XIII. MORBI UNGUIUM

Morbi, qui ungues infestare solent, sunt:

Seline

Est macula alba in vel sub ungue.

Macula autem albicans in radice unguis conspicua *lunula unguis* dicitur.

Species sunt :

I. **Seline a carie sicca unguium**, quae vitri acuti fragmento tam diu radi debet, donec macula dispareat. Subinde spiritus vini camphoratus conducit.

2. **Seline a pustula sub ungue**, quae rasuram unguis cum cultro exigit, ut pus exire possit.

~~~~~~~~~~

Ecchymoma Unguis

Est macula livida sub ungue.

Species sunt:

1. **Ecchymoma violentum**, quod a contusione, pressura, acupunctura unguis vel festuca sub unguem intrusa oritur.

Curatur fomento calido ex oxycrato vel vino.

2. **Ecchymoma a frigore aeris**. Evanescit in calore.
~~~~~~~~~~

CLASS XIII. DISEASES OF THE NAIL

Diseases that usually invade the nails are:

Seline [leukonychia]

Seline is a white spot on or under the nail. However, the whitish spot clearly visible in the root of the nail is called the lunula of the nail.

The species are:

1. **Seline a carie sicca unguium** [leukonychia from dry corruption of the nail], which should be scraped with a sharp piece of glass for as long as necessary until the spot disappears. Sometimes camphorated spirit of wine is helpful.

2. **Seline a pustula sub ungue** [leukonychia from pustule under the nail], which requires the scraping of the nail with a knife so that pus is able to come out.

~~~~~~~~~~

Ecchymoma Unguis [bruised nails]

Ecchymoma unguis is a bluish spot under the nail.

The species are:

1. **Ecchymoma violentum** [traumatic bruised nails, subungual hematoma], which arises from a contusion, pressure, puncture of the nail with a needle, or from a splinter intruded under the nail.

It is treated with a warm compress made from oxycrate or wine.

2. **Ecchymoma a frigore aeris** [bruised nails from cold air]. Disappears in heat.
~~~~~~~~~~

3. **Ecchymoma a frigore febrili**. Est livor unguium in stadio frigoris febrilis. Evanescit in stadio caloris.

4. **Ecchymoma trihomaticum** [*sic*]. Ante eruptionem trichomatis aliquando omnes ungues nigerrimi fiunt, & abscedunt.

~~~~~~~~~~

Gryphosis

Est unguium, postquam longe excreverunt, incurvatio.

Species sunt:

1. **Gryphosis a neglecta abscissione**.[1] Curatio exigit abscissionem ope foricipis scindentis vel serrula, si unguis nimis durus.

2. **Gryphosis a resecta plica polonica**. Inter alia symptomata potissimum unguium excrescentia mirabilis, cum scabritie & nigredine, ut ungues cornua hircina referant, observatur.

Curatio exigit ablationem trichomatis.

3. **Gryphosis anonyma** seu a morbo ignoto.[2]

[1] Hominibus, quoties ungues vel ex barbarie vel ex more aliquo antiquo omittunt resecare, ad 3 & 4 pollices & spithamam longi fiunt. Haller *Physiol.* T. V. p. 30. Cel. Camper *Abh. von Schuh.* pag. 56. unguem pollicis majoris, qui super omnes reliquos digitos pedis excrescebat, adhucdum conservat inter sua praeparata anatomico-pathologica.

[2] Ex morbo duos pollices longos ungues Lindenius *in sua physiologia* refert. Duas uncias longos in *Phil. Trans.* n. 297. quatuor cum dimidio Jacobaeus conf. Bartuolini *anat.* p. 57.

~~~~~~~~~~

3. **Ecchymoma a frigore febrile** [bruised nails from cold fever]. It is a bluish discoloration of the nails in the stage of cold fever. It disappears in the stage of warm fever.

4. **Ecchymoma trichomaticum** [trichoma-associated bruised nails]. Before the development of trichoma, sometimes all the nails become very black and slough off.

~~~~~~~~~~

Gryphosis [onychogryphosis]

Gryphosis is the inward curve of a nail after it has grown a long way out.

The species are:

1. **Gryphosis a neglecta abscissione**[1] [gryphosis from neglecting to cut]. The treatment requires cutting away the nail with the help of cutting forceps or a small saw if the nail is too hard.

2. **Gryphosis a resecta plica polonica** [gryphosis from a resected plica polonica]. Among other symptoms, in particular, the wondrous overgrowth of the nails is observed, with roughness and blackening, resulting in nails that bring to mind goat-like horns.

Treatment requires removal of the trichoma.

3. **Gryphosis anonyma**[gryphosis without a name] or from an unknown disease.[2]

[1] In men, whenever they neglect to trim their nails either from barbarism or from some old custom, they become a length as long as 3–4 thumbs (2.91–3.88 inches). Haller's *Elements of Physiology*. Book V, p. 30. The celebrated Peter Camper's *Treatise on the Best Form of Shoes*, p. 56, still preserves among his anatomic-pathologic preparations a nail of the great toe that was growing out above all the remaining digits of his foot.

[2] Lindenius reports in his physiology nails two thumbs (1.938 inches) long from the disease. *Philosophical Transactions* reports nails 2 inches long on page 297; Jacobaeus reports a nail 4.5 inches long. Compare Bartuolini's Anatomy, page 57.

~~~~~~~~~~

Fissura Unguium

Est unguis solutio lineam referens.

Species sunt:

1. **Fissura cruenta**, quae ab instrumento acuto infligitur, & unione ut vulnus curatur.

2. **Fissura sicca**, quae sua sponte subinde observatur, aliquando autem luis venereae vel leprae effectus est.

Curatio instituatur juxta morbum, a quo fissura pendet.

~~~~~~~~~~

Tinea Unguium

Est unguis unius, vel plurium erosio seu corruptio ulcerosa. Species sunt:

1. **Tinea sicca**, V. *Scabrities unguium.*

2. **Tinea humida**, in qua unguis mollis rugosus, hinc inde corruptus & saniosus est.

Causa proxima est depositio humoris acris, qui circa radicem unguis deponitur.

Id contingit in lue venerea, in impetigine, in plica polonica, in lepra & elephantiasi.

Curatio exigit, ut acrimonia suo specifico remedio auferatur.

Externe spiritus vini camphoratus cum mastiche prodest.
~~~~~~~~~~

Fissura Unguium [fissured nail]

Fissura unguium refers to the weakening of a nail with a linear split.

The species are:

1. **Fissura cruenta** [bloody fissure], which is inflicted by a sharp instrument, and it is cured with closure as a wound.

2. **Fissura sicca** [dry fissure], which is frequently observed to be spontaneous but is sometimes brought about by lues venerea or lepra.

The treatment should be instituted according to the underlying disease on which the fissure depends.

~~~~~~~~~~

Tinea Unguium [tinea of the nail]

Tinea unguium is an ulcerous erosion or corruption of one or more nails. The species are:

1. **Tinea sicca** [dry tinea], see *Scabrities unguium.*

2. **Tinea humida** [wet tinea], in which the nail is soft, wrinkled, and here and there corrupted and bloody.

The proximate cause is the depositing of a pungent humor, positioned around the root of the nail.

This happens in lues venerea, impetigo, plica polonica (see next class), lepra, and elephantiasis.

The treatment requires that the acrimony be taken away by its own specific remedy.

Externally, the camphorated spirit of wine with mastiche is beneficial.
~~~~~~~~~~

Mollities Unguium

Est unguium tanta flexilitas, ut sine ruptura plicari, & corrugari possint. Hic morbus subinde a tinea unguium, subinde a chlorosi oritur.

Curatio. Mollities *tineosa* ut tinea unguis, mollities *chlorotica* martialibus curatur.[1]

[1] Nieman. [*sic*] *Dissertatio epistolica de foeda unguium mollitie puellae chloroticae martialium usu feliciter curate.* Magdeberg. 1774.

~~~~~~~~~~

Scabrities Unguium

Est unguium sicca, quasi cariosa corruptio, qua unguis scaber, crassus, friabilis & inaequalis evadit.

Hic morbus etiam *tinea sicca* unguium vocari potest; subinde solam radicem, vel solum marginem adhaesivum, subinde totum unguem occupat.

Oritur a valido labore, quo radix ungis [*sic*] vitiatur, aliquando etiam a causa interna nascitur.

Curatio exigit, ut frustum lardi corrupto ungui per aliquot septimanas firmiter applicetur.

Pterigium Unguis

Est epidermidis magna prolongatio & incrementum supra radices unguium.

Curatio exigit, ut epidermis obtuso cultro ab ungue separetur & reprimatur.

Ulcera circa marginem unguis frequenter *carnem fungosam*, quae supra unguem proserpere videtur, formare solent. Haec lapide infernali auferatur, & dein aqua cum aqua vulneraria ex cortice peruviano, aqua Thediana & extracto saturni parata exsiccetur.

~~~~~~~~~~

Mollities Unguium [soft nails]

Mollities unguium is such great flexibility of the nails that they are able to be folded over without breaking and able to be wrinkled. This disease sometimes arises from tinea unguium, sometimes from chlorosis.

Treatment. Mollities *tineosa* is treated as tinea unguium; mollities *chlorotica* is treated with medicinal iron preparations.[1]

[1] Johann Christoph Niemann. *Epistolary dissertation about the ugliness of a soft nail of a chlorotic girl that was happily cured with the use of martial water.* Magdeburg. 1774

~~~~~~~~~~

Scabrities Unguium [dry nails]

Scabrities unguium is the dryness of the nails as if decayed from corruption, which gives way to a scabby, thick, friable, and uneven nail.

This disease can also be called *tinea sicca* of the nails. It sometimes adheres to only the base of the nail, or to only the margin, or sometimes to the entire nail.

It arises from manual labor by which the root of the nail is damaged; occasionally, it is even born from an internal cause.

The treatment requires that a scrap of bacon be applied firmly to the corrupted nail for several weeks.

Pterigium Unguis [wing-shaped nails]

Pterigium unguis is a large elongation and increase of epidermis over the root of the nail.

The treatment requires that the epidermis be divided and pressed back with a blunt knife.

Ulcers around the margin of the nail frequently form *exophytic flesh*, which appears to creep forward over the nail. These may be taken away with *lapis infernalis*, and next dried up with water prepared with *aqua vulneraria* from Peruvian bark, Thedian water, and Saturnine extract.

~~~~~~~~~~

Arctura Unguis

Est unguis curvatura lateralis, cutem secans & exulcerans.

Noscitur inflammatione, dolore intenso & exulceratione laterali digiti, praesertim pollicis majoris in pede.

Oritur ab excisione nimis acuta marginis lateralis in ungue aut a calceis nimium angustis.

Curatio exigit, ut unguis medietas fragmento acuto vitri tamdiu fricetur, donec margo lateralis sursum pergat; sub unguem ponitur linteum carptum, & ad ulcus applicetur extractum saturni, aqua dilutum, vel aqua vulneraria viridis[1] vel aqua vulneraria chinata.[2]

Si haec medicatio non juvat, discindatur forfice acutissima unguis a margine usque ad radicem, dein portio unguis carni increta, forcipe evellator.

[1] Ill. Baldinger neues *Magazin für Aerzte.* 3. B. I. p. 26. vom *Nagelgeschwür.* Rx. vini albi ℔ij. viridis aeris, aluminis aa ℥ß, mellis ℥ß. m. coquantur leniter.

[2] Ego sequantem aquam centies egregiam sum expertus. Rx. Aquae fontanae ℥viij. Aquae Thedianae ℥iij. Extract saturni. Salis ammoniaci aa ʒß. Cort. peruviana ℥j m. f. aqua.

~~~~~~~~~~

Deformitas Unguis

Est unguium monstrosum incrementum in formam unguiculae avicularis vel cornu.[1]

Curatio exigit abscissionem.

[1] Historiam unguium, qui in vera cornua laminata abierunt, V. in *Histoir. de l'Academ.* 1719. hist. I. Hominem quotidie coram me video, qui sibi digitum auricularem manus sinistrae in sua juventute intra portam adeo compresserat, ut totus unguis ablatus fuerit, renascebatur loco unguis cornu acutum, quod unguis substantiam habet, admodum crassum & longum fit, si non omni mense refecetur.
~~~~~~~~~~

Arctura Unguis [ingrown nail]

Arctura unguis is a nail with lateral curvature, cutting and ulcerating on the skin.

It is recognized by inflammation, intense pain, and ulceration of the side of the digit, especially of the big toe.

It arises from cutting too sharply to a point the lateral nail margin or from wearing shoes that are too narrow.

The treatment requires that the middle of the nail be rubbed with a sharp fragment of glass for as long as it takes, where the lateral margin continues upward, under the nail is placed lint from flax, and to the wound should be applied Saturn extract diluted with water or *aqua vulneraria viridis*[1] or *aqua vulneraria chinata*.[2]

If this medication does not help, separate with very sharp scissors the nail from the edge all the way to the root, then the portion of the nail that has grown into the flesh should be plucked off with forceps.

[1] The illustrious Ernst Gottfried Baldinger in *New Magazine for Doctors*, Volume 3, Book 1, p. 26. *On Paronychia*. Rx. ½ oz. each of green copper and alum and honey should be cooked gently in 2 pounds weight of white wine.

[2] I have experience with the following excellent water over 100 times: 8 oz. of spring water, 3 oz. of Thedian water, ½ dram each of lead acetate and ammonium salt, 1 oz. of Peruvian bark. Let it be mixed in water.

~~~~~~~~~~

Deformitas Unguis [deformed nail]

Deformitas unguis is a monstrous growth of nails in the shape of a bird's claw or a horn.[1]

Treatment requires cutting it away.

[1] See the case history of nails that have transformed into true, thin-plated horns in *History of the Academy*, 1719. Case 1. I myself see a man every day who in his youth had so greatly compressed the <u>ear finger</u> of his left hand in a gate that the entire nail had been torn off; in the place of a nail a sharp horn arose that has the substance of a nail, and it becomes very long and thick if not cut away every month.
~~~~~~~~~~

Lapsus Unguium

Est unguis unius vel plurium spontaneus secessus a digito.

Causae, quae hunc lapsum efficiunt, sunt suppuratio sub vel circa radicem unguis, longa manuum maceratio in aqua calida, virus plicosum, vel aliud, & datum venenum.

A lapsu unguis ad minimum loci denudati attactum fiunt horrendi dolores.

Curatio requirit, ut inspergatur ad locum ab ungue nudum pulvis olibani vel mastichis, & molli cera, quae unguis figuram referat, tegatur.

Sic unguis a sua radice incipit iterum crescere, & restitui.

Lapsus Unguium [onycholysis]

Lapsus unguium is the spontaneous shedding of one or more nails from its digit.

The causes that bring about this separation are suppuration under or around the base of the nail, prolonged soaking of the hands in warm water, the plica virus or some other virus, or from being given poison.

Terrible pains from lapsus unguium occur with the slightest contact with the denuded part.

Treatment requires that the place separated from the nail be sprinkled with frankincense powder or mastiche, and covered with soft wax, which mimics the shape of the nail.

Thus the nail begins to grow again from its root and be restored.

CLASSIS XIV. MORBI PILORUM

Morbos, qui pilos afficiunt, ut morbos unguium ad cutaneos refero, cum ungues & pili partes cutis esse censeantur.

Sunt autem *morbi pilorum* sequentes.

Calvities

Est pilorum in capite vel alia parte crinita defectus.[1]

Causa proxima est osculorum in bulbis, quae pilos emittunt, nimia amplitudo, vel nimia arctitudo seu concretio vel bulbuli ipsius morbositas.

Dividitur generatim calvities:

In *universalem*, si totum caput calvum glabrumque sit.
In *partialem*: si quidam tantum capillatae partis locus capillis careat. Haec species dicitur *Area* seu *Alopectia* [*sic*], si locus depilis plagam: *Ophiasis* si locus calvus serpentem ab occipitio, ad frontem vel utrinque ad tempora pergentem referat. Datur demum calvities barbae, axillarum, pubis, oculorum.

Species sunt:

1. **Calvities febrisequa**, quae febres acutas sequitur.

2. **Calvities puerperarum**. Quibusdam mulieribus in omni puerperio plus minus defluunt capilli.

3. **Calvities morborum exanthematicorum**. Variolas aut erysipelas saepe calvities sequitur.

4. **Calvities acrimoniosa**. Huc pertinet calvities a praegressa tinea, achoribus, trichomate, lepra, lue venerea, scorbuto &c.

CLASS XIV. DISEASES OF THE HAIR

I refer to diseases as cutaneous that affect the hair, as I do the diseases of the nails, since the nails and hair are considered to be parts of the skin.

However, the following are *diseases of the hair*:

Calvities [hair loss]

Calvities is the disappearance of hair on the head or other hairy area.[1]

The proximate cause is that the openings in the follicle, which put forth the hairs, are too wide, or too narrow, or compacted, or if the follicle itself is unhealthy.

Calvities is generally divided:

> into *universal*, if the whole head is bald and smooth;
> into *partial*, if only some portion of the scalp is lacking hairs. This species is called *area* or *alopectia* [*sic*], if the site of hair loss is a region; *ophiasis* is the term if the bald spot mimics a serpent crawling away from the occiput, to the forehead or progressing from either or both sides to the temples. Finally given is calvities of the head, underarms, pubic area, and eyes.

The species are:

1. **Calvities febrisequa** [hair loss after fever/telogen effluvium], which follows acute fevers.

2. **Calvities puerperarum** [postpartum hair loss/telogen effluvium]. Some women shed more or less hair in each childbirth period.

3. **Calvities morborum exanthematicorum** [hair loss of exanthematous disease/telogen effluvium]. Hair loss often follows smallpox or erysipelas.

4. **Calvities acrimoniosa** [acrimonious hair loss]. This pertains to calvities from prior tinea, achor, trichoma, lepra, syphilis, scurvy, etc.

5. **Calvities phthisicorum**. Est capillorum defluvium, quod in consumata phthisi vel hectica observatur.

6. **Calvities a debilitate nervosa**: terror, veneris abusus, magna animi per curas agitatio, cephalaea induxere calvitiem.[2]

7. **Calvities senum** est naturalis capillorum defectus in syncipite & vertice senum.

8. **Calvities haereditaria**. Quae multis familiis jam in aetate juvenili vel virili consueta est. In Insula Mycono infantes calvi dicuntur nasci vel 20 anno jam calvescunt.[3]

9. **Calvities a vapore mercurii**, quae in aurifabris quandoque observatur, & diaeta lactea curata fuit.

10. **Calvities a causa externa**: ut a dropace, a mitra aspera &c.

Prognosis. Si locus calvus frictione non rubeat, tunc calvities incurabilis censetur.[5] Senilis nunquam, hereditaria & inveterata, ut & universalis raro curatur. Palingenesia crinium quandoque diversi a prioribus coloris & figurae est.

Curatio exigit, ut causa materialis calvitiei tollatur, dein ut oscula pilos emittentia nimis laxa roborantibus arctentur, nimis arcta relaxentur, impervia autem ope rasurae referantur. Hinc praemissis catharticis antacrimoniosa, vel roborantia vel in siccitate humectantia interne dentur.

Externe specifice laudantur: rasura capitis, aqua stillatitia e favis apum, axungia ursi, lixivium cinerum, in quo hedera arborea vel malvae radix vel buxus[6] infusus aut coctus, succus caeparum affrictus, ladanum oleo solutum, succus tabaci, thapsiae ʒj cum axungiae ursi ℥j in unquentum [*sic*] redacta.

[1] D. Pfeiffer *diss. de calvitie*. Budae 1783. Calvities Graecis *φαλάκρωσις*, vel *Madarosis* dicitur.

5. **Calvities phthisicorum** [hair loss of tuberculosis]. This is shedding of hair, which is observed in consumption or hectic fever.

6. **Calvities a debilitate nervosa** [hair loss from nervous disorder]: terror, sexual abuse, great agitation of spirit because of worry, and headache induce hair loss.[2]

7. **Calvities senum** [hair loss of old men; male pattern hair loss] is natural loss of the hair on the frontal scalp and vertex.

8. **Calvities haereditaria** [hereditary hair loss], which is not unusual for many families even in the time of youth or early adulthood. On the island of Mykonos, infants are said to be born bald or are already bald by 20 years of age.[3]

9. **Calvities a vapore mercurii** [hair loss from mercury vapor], which is sometimes observed in goldsmiths and has been cured with a milky diet.[4]

10. **Calvities a causa externa** [hair loss from an external cause]: as from a depilatory or rough headband, etc.

Prognosis. If the bald spot does not redden with friction, then the calvities is considered incurable.[5] The geriatric, hereditary, and chronic types are never cured, and the universal type is rarely cured. Regrowth of hair sometimes is different from previous in color and quality.

Treatment requires that the material cause of the calvities be removed, then that the pores emitting the hairs that are too loose be compressed with reinforcement; the ones that are compressed should be relaxed, but the compacted should be restored with the help of a razor. At this point, previously mentioned anti-acrimonious cathartics, either strengthening or moistening for the dryness, should be given internally.

Externally are specifically praised: shaving of the head; water drops from the honeycombs of bees; bear lard; solution of ash, in which is infused or boiled tree ivy or mallow root or boxwood;[6] juice of a rubbed onion, rockrose oil solution, tobacco juice, 1 dram thapsia with 1 oz. bear lard rendered in unguent.

[1] Lajos Pfeiffer *Dissertation on Calvities.* Budae, 1783. Calvities is called by the Greeks *phalacrosis* or *madarosis.*

[2] Exempla de his omnibus collegit D. Pfeiffer. l. c. p. 14

[3] Tournefort *vog. en lev.* T. I. p. 333.

[4] Foresti *observ. & curat.* L. 8. obs. 5.

[5] Zacuti *Prax. histor.* L. 7. C. I. p. 5.

[6] *Misc. N. C.* dec. 2. ann. 2. obs. 155. lixivio buxi incautius faciem & collum lotum non tantum in capite loto sed etiam in facie & collo copiose progerminasse fertur.

~~~~~~~~~~

Hirsuties

Est pilorum exortus nimius, vel in toto corpore vel in loco non consueto.

Causa proxima est bulborum progenies in loco non consueto vel affluxus nimius nutrimenti ad bulbos pilorum.

Nascuntur subinde foetus adeo hirsuti, ut pro simiis habiti fuerint. Huc etiam refero feminas barbatas & duplicia supercilia super uno oculo.

Hirsuties ergo vel *universalis* in tota corporis superficie est, vel *partialis* in uno tantum vel consueto vel inconsueto loco.[1]

Curatio. Applicetur spiritus salis dulcis, qui mediante charta bibula apponitur, vel unguentum depilatorium ex auripigmento, calce viva & melle.

[1] Homo ex sua natura hirsutum est animal, totum pilis adspersum, si volam manus, plantam pedis, & penis glandem excipias, nam etiam in facie & mammis formosissimae feminae pili deprehenduntur. Quoties jam hi pili, qui vulgo breves manent in homine, in aliqualem longitudinem excrescunt, tunc homines *hirsuti* seu *pilosi* vocantur. Foetus aliquando toti pilosi nascuntur, feminae barbatae & homines in tota facie pilosi fuere visi. In ovarii, aliarumque partium atheromatibus frequenter pili crispi & alii inveniuntur. Sic etiam in omento, in ventriculo pili effloruerunt, lingua non raro pilosa evadit. Pilam
~~~~~~~~~~

[2] Lajos Pfeiffer collected examples of all of these in the previous citation, p. 14.

[3] *A Voyage into the Levant*, by Joseph Pitton de Tournefort. Book 1. p. 333.

[4] Petrus Forestus *Observations and Cures*. Book 8. Observation 5.

[5] Abraham Zacutus. *Praxis historiarum*. Book 7. Chapter 1. p. 5.

[6] *Miscellaneous Natural Curiosities*. Division 2. Year 2. Observation 155. Having rather incautiously washed the face and neck with lye of boxwood, it is said to have brought forth hair copiously, not only on the washed head, but also on the face and neck.

~~~~~~~~~~

Hirsuties [hirsutism]

Hirsuties is the growth of excessive hair, either on the entire body or in an unaccustomed place.

The proximate cause is the progeny of bulbous roots in an unaccustomed place or the overflow of excessive nutrients to the bulbs of hairs.

Fetuses are occasionally born with such hirsuties that they have been regarded as monkeys. I also make reference here to bearded women and the double eyebrows above one eye.

Hirsuties, therefore, is either *universal* on the entire surface of the body or *partial* in only one accustomed or unaccustomed location.[1]

Treatment. Sweet spirit of salt which should be applied by means of blotting paper, or depilatory ointment from auripigment, quicklime, and honey.

[1] Man by his nature is a hairy animal, completely covered by hair, if you exempt the palm of the hand, the sole of the foot, and glans of the penis, for hair is even discerned on the face and breasts of the most beautiful women. Whenever these hairs which usually remain short in man grow out to a large extent, then men are called *hairy* or *shaggy*. Fetuses are sometimes born completely hairy, bearded women have been seen, and men seen with hair over their whole face. In cysts of the ovaries and of other parts, curled hair and other things are frequently found. In such a manner, hair has also flourished
~~~~~~~~~~

capillorum super musculum rectum abdominis, & in carne bubula folliculum, in quo intricati pili erant, descripserunt Authores. V. III. Halleri *elementa Physiologicae* T. V. p. 32 & 33.

~~~~~~~~~~

Xerasia

Est capillorum nimia tenuitas, lanugini similis.

Curatio exigit, ut caput novacula abradatur, & saepius unguento pomato inungatur, atque pulvere cyprio inspergatur. Decoctum buxi denique tentandum.

~~~~~~~~~~

Trichoma seu Plica Polonica

Est praeternaturalis pilorum in quacunque pilosa corporis parte in funiculos vel pannos intricatio,[1] nulla arte humana extricabilis.

Dividitur plica.

> In *cirrosam*, quae plica *mas* vocatur, dum unus vel plures cirri contorti e parte crinita instar caudarum glirium pendent.
>
> In villosam, quae plica *femina* dicitur, dum omnes fere crines in se mutuo intertexti speciem pilei villosi seu mitrae vel panni cujusdam rigidi efformant.

Sedes. Caput capillatum plerumque huic malo obnoxium est, tamen etiam in barba, & in pube visa est plica. Brutis e juba aut cauda erumpit. Longitudo ejusdem quandoque enormis est.

Causa proxima est peculiare miasma, quod uberiorem & criticum secessum succi crines nutrientis causat. Indoles atque origo hujus miasmatis adhuc ignoratur. Hoc miasma ex India orientali circa annum 1687 per Tartaros in Poloniam, Silesiam, Hungariam, Sarmatiam, Russiam, & loca vicina invectum fuisse creditur. In aliis regionibus vix conspicuus est morbus.

in the bowels and in the stomach, and not infrequently the tongue becomes hairy. The authors have described a ball of hair above the rectus abdominis, and a small sac in the meat of cattle, in which hairs were ensnared. See the illustrious Haller *Elements of Physiology* Book 5, pp 32 & 33.

~~~~~~~~~~

Xerasia [fine hair]

Xerasia is an extreme thinness of hair, similar to lanugo hairs.

The treatment requires that the head be abraded with a razor, and anointed quite often with pomade ointment and also sprinkled with cyprus powder. Finally, boiled boxwood ought to be tried.

~~~~~~~~~~

Trichoma or Plica Polonica

Trichoma or plica polonica is an unnatural entanglement of hairs in cords or matted on any hairy part of the body,[1] and it is not humanly possible to untangle it.

Plica is divided:

> into *cirrosa*, which is called male plica, when one or more contorted curls hang from the hairy part with the appearance of the tails of dormice;
>
> into *villosa*, which is called female plica, when nearly all hairs—having mutually interwoven with each other—form the appearance of a shaggy cap, turban, or some sort of stiff cloth.

Seats. In general, the scalp hair is vulnerable to this malady; however, plica has even been seen in the beard and pubic area. It erupts like an animal's mane or tail. The length of it is sometimes enormous.

The proximate cause is a particular miasma that causes a rather productive and critical withdrawal of juice nourishing the hairs. The nature and origin of this miasma is yet unknown. This miasma is believed to have been carried by the Tartars from eastern India about the year 1687 into Poland, Silesia, Hungary, Sarmatia, Russia, and neighboring places. In other regions, the disease is scarcely seen.

Morbi contagium *nativitate* a parentibus trichomatosis, vel concubitu cum homine infecto vel usu lecti, vestimentive miasmate infecti, communicatur.

Species sunt:

1. **Trichoma latens seu occultum**. Ante plicae eruptionem per plures menses atrocissimus capitis dolor adest cum sudore viscido crinium, noctu molesto, copiosisque furfuribus locum plicae, ubi erumpit, conspurcantibus. Arthritis vaga & fixa, pleuritis; cardialgia, colica, oedema crurum, glandularum infarctus tubercula cutanea, tophi arthritici, ulcera oris, narium, viscerum febres variae auctae & intermittentes, deliria acuta & chronica, convulsiones, spasmi, paralyses, paretes, alvi fluxus, haemorrhagiae, oculorum varii morbi, ophthalmia, amaurosis, dolor, pica, ungues scabri, lividi, recurvi, corrupti, quandoque humores pilosi sub cute cranii latentes.[2]

2. **Trichoma evolutum**. Critica plicae excretio per longum tempus durat, perfecta cognoscitur fuga omnium symptomatum, capillorum defluvio, qui dein resarciuntur.

3. **Trichoma suppressum.** A resecta ante perfectam crisim plica, iidem oriuntur morbi, quos in latente trichomate adnotavimus, qui redeunte plica iterum evanescunt. Tolluntur hi morbi:

    1. Plicae spontanea *eruptione.*
    2. *Phthiriasi* cum porrigine, & *sudore* foetido capitis.
    3. *Alopecia* spontanea.
    4. Datis medicamentis specificis contra plicam.

4. **Trichoma spurium**. Est capillorum intricatio, quae a neglecta pectinatione & sordida porrigine capitis nascitur.[3] Absentia symptomatum in trichomate vero consuetorum cognoscitur.

Curatur resectione capillorum & purificatione capitis. V. *Achores.*

The contagium of the disease is spread at *birth* from trichomatis parents, or by intercourse with an infected person, or using a bed or clothing infected with the miasma.

The species are:

1. **Trichoma latens or occultum** [latent trichoma]. Before the eruption of plica, the most atrocious pain in the head is present for several months, with a slimy sweat of hairs, troublesome at night, and copious furfur polluting the site of the plica where it erupts. Both wandering and fixed arthritis, pleurisy, chest pain, colic, leg edema, blocked glands, cutaneous nodules, arthritic tophi, ulcers of the mouth, nares, and intestinal tract, fevers that are intermittent and varying in intensity, acute and chronic delirium, convulsions, spasms, paralysis, paresis, diarrhea, hemorrhages, various diseases of the eyes, ophthalmia, amaurosis, pain, pica, scabby, livid, curved, corrupted nails, sometimes hairy humors lying hidden under the skin of the head.[2]

2. **Trichoma evolutum** [evolved trichoma]. The relevant excretion of plica lasts for a long time; the complete resolution of all symptoms is experienced with the shedding of hairs, which are then restored.

3. **Trichoma suppressum** [suppressed trichoma]. By resecting the plica before it achieves its critical stage, the same diseases arise which we have observed in latent trichoma, and then disappear when the plica returns again. These diseases of latent trichoma are removed with:

    1. spontaneous eruption of plica.

    2. lice with porrigo and fetid sweat of the scalp.

    3. spontaneous alopecia.

    4. by giving specific medicaments against the plica.

4. **Trichoma spurium** [false trichoma]. It is the interweaving of hair, which develops from neglected brushing and dirty scalp porrigo.[3] It is recognized by the absence of symptoms typical of true trichoma.

It is treated with resection of the hairs and cleansing of the scalp. See *Achor.*

Curatio. Cum antidotum hujus miasmatis adhuc desideretur, necesse est.

1. Ut *latens* miasma excernatur:

2. - *excretum* non repellatur, aut

3. - *retropulsum* iterum in capillitium revocetur.

Latens miasma ad excretionem invitatur 1. Ope fomentorum calidorum, capillitio capitis diu applicatorum. Optimum est caput decocto lycopodii bis de die lavare, vel unguento lycopodii, bis de die illinere.[4] Arnicae aut roris marini flores in aqua vel cerevisia cocti, specifice ad hunc scopum laudantur. 2. *Interne* idem decoctum lycopodii vel infusum arnicae, aut rorismarini[5] [*sic*] cum sale succini, aut viperarum tamdiu exhibetur, donec symptomata remittant & plica prodeat.

In casu graviori adhibentur vesicatoria ad nucham, theriaca, tinctura metallorum, pulvis ex sulphure aurato antimonii, & camphora. Decoctum sarsaparillae & radicis serpentariae virginianae. Unguibus apponatur cera rubra mollis ad sigillandum usualis.

Purgantia valentiora, emetica, mercurialia, nitrosa copiose data, atque venaesectio morbum valde exasperant. Rescissio plicae & capillorum est summe exitialis, cum pessimi exinde morbi subsequantur. Sed spontaneus plicae delapsus, qui vero admodum raro contingit, subinde salutaris fuit.[6]

[1] Vide egregiam *diss.* D. Gabriel *de Plica polonica.* Budae. 1780. & Cel. Vicat *Memoires sur la plique polonoise.*

[2] Gabriel *l. c.* p. 21.

[3] Cel. Vicat *l. c.* p. 46.

[4] Gabriel *l. c.* p. 78.

[5] Hebraeo plica polonica laboranti infuso rorismarini [*sic*] arthritidem & cephalaeam nuper curavi, plica etiam emendabatur, at aegrotus paullo post aufugiebat.

Treatment. Since an antidote to this miasma is still greatly wished for, it is necessary that:

1. the *latent* miasma be excreted;

2. the *excretion* must not be forced back inward, so that,

3. the previously *driven out* miasma will not be called back into the hair.

Latent miasma is induced to excretion 1. with the help of warm compresses, applied to the hair for a long time. It is best to wash the head with a lycopodium decoction twice a day, or to anoint with lycopodium unguent twice a day.[4] Flowers of arnica or rosemary boiled in water or beer are praised specifically for this purpose. 2. Likewise, a decoction of lycopodium, or infusion of arnica, or of rosemary with salt of amber,[5] or of vipers, is given internally the whole time until the symptoms subside and the plica comes out.

In a more serious case, vesicatories are employed for the nape of the neck, along with theriac, tincture of metals, powder from golden sulfur of antimony, and camphor. A decoction of sarsaparilla and Virginia snakeroot [is also employed]. Soft red wax, as used for sealing, should be applied with the fingernails to the scalp.

Relatively strong purgatives, emetics, mercurials, copious amounts of saltpeter, and bloodletting greatly provoke the disease. Cutting the plica and hair is extremely deadly, since very bad diseases follow immediately afterward. But when the plica falls off spontaneously, which indeed occurs very rarely, it has sometimes been beneficial.[6]

[1] See the excellent *dissertation from* Gabriel *de Plica polonica*. Budae. 1780 & the celebrated B.B.Vicat's *Dissertation on the Polish plica*.

[2] Ibid, p. 21.

[3] Vicat, p. 46.

[4] Gabriel, p. 78.

[5] I have recently cured with an infusion of rosemary the arthritis and continuous headache of a Jewish patient suffering from plica polonica. The plica was also improved, but the sick man soon after vanished.

[6] Interim tamen tonsio capitis aliquando utilis fuit. De plica valde immunda tonsione capitis sanata observationem habet Trioen v. ejus *observationes. Cl. Prof. Pragensis* Mikan curavit feminae, jam a multis annis plicosae, capillos abscindi; altero die enormis capitis dolor, vertigo & debilitas sequuntur, mnlta [sic] remedia gratis tentantur, omnia in pejus ruunt, demum capilli penitus abraduntur, & sic haec faemina integre convaluit.

~~~~~~~~~~

Fissura Capillorum

Est spontanea dehiscentia capillorum in duo vel plura filamenta.[1] Rarissime vel nunquam ad cutem usque capilli finduntur, sed tantummodo in fine extremo.

Causa proxima est capillorum aridura, vel vitiosus succus, vel abundantia succi capillaris. Hinc capilli fissi saepe defluunt.

Curatio exigit, ut capitiluvia ex herbis aromaticis & recens unguentum pomatum adhibeatur. *Interne* dentur, quae sanguinem purificant.

[1] Graecis hic morbus dicitur *Dichophyia*

~~~~~~~~~~

Canities

Est coloris capillorum mutatio in album vel gryseum colorem. Causa proxima esse videtur exsiccatio seu aridura bulborum capillarium.[1]

Species sunt:

1. **Canities senilis**, quae senectutis est naturalis effectus. Quibus venerabile hoc senectutis ornamentum displicet, hi caput suum caesarie adscititia tegere, aut frequenti pectinatione cum pectine plumbeo colorem nigrum inducere tenentur. Sunt demum, qui cum solutione lapidis infernalis capillos nigricant.

[6] Meanwhile, however, shearing of the head was sometimes useful. Trioen has an observation about a very unclean plica cured by a tonsure of the head. See his observations. The *celebrated Professor* Mikan of *Prague* treated a woman who had had plica for many years by cutting off her hair; the next day an enormous headache, vertigo, and weakness followed. Many remedies were tried without reward; everything made it worse. Finally, the hair was completely shaved off, and thus this woman fully recovered.

~~~~~~~~~~

Fissura Capillorum [split hairs, trichoptilosis]

Fissura capillorum is the spontaneous splitting of the hairs into two or more filaments.[1] Very rarely or never are the hairs cleaved all the way to the skin, but they are nearly split at the very end of the hairs.

The proximate cause is dryness of the hair, or corrupt moisture, or abundance of moisture in the hair. From these causes, the split hairs often fall out.

The treatment requires that shampoo from aromatic herbs and fresh pomade unguent be applied. Internally, those things which purify the blood should be given.

[1] This disease is called *Dichophyia* by the Greeks.

~~~~~~~~~~

Canities [graying of hair]

Canities is the change in color of the hair to a white or gray color. The proximate cause seems to be a drying up or a parched condition of the bulbs of the hairs.[1]

The species are:

1. **Canities senilis** [senile graying] is a natural effect of old age. For those to whom this venerable ornament of old age is displeasing, they are limited to covering their heads with donated hair or inducing a black color by frequently brushing with a lead comb. There are finally those who blacken their hair with a solution of <u>infernal</u> <u>stone</u>.

2. **Canities praematura**, quae in aetate juvenili vel virili jam contingit. Haec canities saepe hereditaria est, saepe magnum terrorem, aut morbum sequitur.[2] *Tractatur* ut canities senilis.

[1] In senibus, omnibus in regionibus capilli canescunt, cum solus nunc epidermidis color supersit exhausta medulla, a quo color erat, & pellucidi sunt ut vitrum album, dicit Ill. Hallerus, bulbos etiam minores esse ajunt.

[2] Subito aliquos a terrore canuisse multi auctores sunt V. Ill. Halleri *elementa Physiol.* T. V. p. 37.

2. **Canities praematura** [premature graying], already happens by the time of youth or early manhood. This type of canities is often hereditary or often follows great terror or disease.[2] It is managed as canities senilis.

[1] The illustrious Haller says that in old men, the hairs in every area of the scalp turn white, since it is now the only color that remains in the exhausted innermost part of the epidermis, from which the color [of the hair] came. They are transparent as white glass, and they say that the bulb roots are even smaller.

[2] Many authors have reported that some people have hairs that suddenly turned white from terror. See Haller's *Elements of Physiology*.

CONCLUSION

Doctrina de Morbis Cutaneis is a true eighteenth-century *vade mecum*, a quick reference for differential diagnosis and treatment options, prepared according to Plenck "for the sake of easier understanding." The work contains only the most essential and pertinent information; yet, it is comprehensive at the same time. Plenck spared his reader the rambling commentary on theory that was so typical of sixteenth-to-eighteenth-century medical treatises. The translation reveals a surprisingly sweeping overview of many dermatological conditions that are recognizable to the modern dermatologist, and much of the diagnostic information, albeit simplistic, is accurate and applicable today. There are no glaring holes in diagnoses or categories. Plenck had knowledge about skin diseases in both adults and children and frequently mentioned conditions unique to children, such as cradle cap and infantile eczema. Plenck was also cognizant of the geographical distribution of skin diseases, such as Brazilian pemphigus (known today as fogo selvagem) and Asturian lepra (known today as pellagra); thus, his handbook offered a global perspective on skin disease rarely seen at the time.

Plenck's scheme for organizing skin disease is elaborate and contains an unprecedented degree of splitting. The opposite of lumping, splitting refers to breaking down the tree of categorization into as many branches as possible. Every skin book preceding Plenck's demonstrates lumping; thus, the information is less helpful to the modern dermatologist, who is an obligatory splitter. Plenck's scheme is very appealing because achieving precision and accuracy with diagnosis is a critical first step in the practice of dermatology. For example, under "Maculae," Plenck's students could learn about reddish skin conditions in three places: rosacea (9 types), erythema (10 types), and "rubedo cutis" (6 types). He listed twenty-four different types or stages of smallpox. There are eight species of lepra, a term that housed Hansen's disease and several other chronic scaly generalized eruptions, including psoriasis. Plenck had eight types of solitary blisters, eleven types of impetigo, nine types of warty growths, eight types of oral ulcers, eleven nail disorders, and ten types of hair loss. While what can be found in twenty-first-century textbooks of dermatology is even more extensive and "split" than what can be found in Plenck's little book, Plenck deserves high praise for his novel effort to split the information down into as many categories as possible, presumably to improve diagnostic precision in his reader. Plenck's desire to split was a product of his intellectual time period, the Enlightenment.

The language of dermatology (macules, papules, pustules, etc.) still used today originated in this important work, and Plenck was among the first to apply the Linnaean binomial system to naming skin diseases, which is still used in dermatology today, e.g., erythema infectiosum and pityriasis lichenoides. Plenck's use of the binomial system is one of his most lasting contributions and something his critics did not acknowledge.

For a small handbook, the work is strong in its offerings of treatment options, and it is an excellent source for the study of eighteenth-century treatment of skin disease. While there appear to be no groundbreaking discoveries as far as treatments in the text, Plenck offered a concise and specific endorsement of particular treatments out of many known contemporary treatment options. Plenck told his reader which treatments to avoid as often as he recommends which treatments to use. His treatments could be categorized into botanical/herbal, chemical/alchemical/metallic, and purgative. The necessity to purge is mentioned 31 times. It is surprising how infrequently bloodletting is mentioned as a treatment, but the book focuses on chronic diseases, and bloodletting was more commonly used in the acute setting. He advocated mercury (mentioned 41 times in the text) and antimony (10 mentions) in many instances. Externally, baths (25 mentions) and washes are favorites of Plenck, as are various ointments (40 mentions), decoctions (21 mentions), tinctures, and waters. Plenck carefully notes on several occasions the importance of treating diseases of the skin both internally and externally, in keeping with the eighteenth-century belief that external treatments alone could drive morbid material into the body. The idea of treating skin disease locally and without internal treatment did not arrive until the career of Ferdinand von Hebra in the next century. Finally, the work was very up to date for its time in its treatment information; Plenck frequently posted footnotes that reference treatments described in contemporaneous publications.

Plenck's *Doctrina de Morbis Cutaneis* is a trailblazing text for the specialty of dermatology, and if Plenck had had a Bateman-type figure or Kaposi-type figure to follow him, we would all likely be referring to Joseph Jacob Plenck as the "founder of dermatology," not Robert Willan. If only Plenck had been employed by a facility like the Carey Street Dispensary or the Hôpital Saint-Louis, perhaps his legacy would have been more profound. Willan undoubtedly borrowed from Plenck, as claimed by Bateman. The physicians who followed Plenck did not cede any credit to a writer from the previous century, or they risked downplaying their own contributions. *Doctrina* was, first and foremost, a distillation of some very confusing information for students new to the task of tackling skin problems. It was the first attempt to classify skin diseases in a scientific fashion, i.e., by their appearance, and the degree of splitting seen in the resultant system was unprecedented. The most important consideration is that there truly was nothing like it in the history of dermatology that preceded it. It was a groundbreaking, concise, and at the same time comprehensive text that has yet to get the credit it deserves. In an effort to bring order to the chaos of skin disease knowledge for his young pupils, Plenck and his little book unknowingly set dermatology on its path to modernity. For all these reasons, we would like to declare *Doctrina de Morbis Cutaneis* by Joseph Jacob Plenck to be the foundational text for the specialty of dermatology.

GLOSSARY

Acrimony: The presence of substances in the skin that are acrid, that is, bitter and pungent, and which irritate and inflame the skin.

Acrochordon: Skin tag.

Agrimony: A flowering herb believed to have various medicinal properties since ancient times.

Alphos: Obsolete term dating back to ancient times for a skin disease characterized by white depressed macules, long held to be a form of lepra. Morphea, lichen sclerosus, vitiligo, and psoriasis are possible modern counterparts.

Althea: *Hibiscus syriacus*, or the rose of Sharon.

Amaurosis: Sudden transient vision loss in one eye, partial or total blindness due to disease of optic nerve.

Anasarca: Severe generalized edema/swelling of the whole body.

Angelica: *Angelica archangelica*; a medicinal plant of the Apiaceae (celery) family used since the tenth century.

Angina gangrenosa: An obsolete term for acute necrotizing ulcerative gingivitis.

Antibilious meds: Medications that reduce biliousness (excessive bile in the body), typically by a laxative effect.

Antihelminthic: A treatment for worm infestation that either kills the worms or expels them from the body.

Antimony: A metal used in various medicinal preparations during ancient and medieval times. Still used today for leishmaniasis, a parasitic illness.

Antimonial soap: One part of golden antimony sulfide mixed in ten parts of cocoa butter. Later (nineteenth century), it was made by mixing antimony and caustic potash (potassium hydroxide) in Castile soap.

Antiphlogisticum: Medication with anti-inflammatory properties.

Antiscorbutic: A treatment with the potential to treat or prevent scurvy, such as lemon juice.

Apoplexy: An old term for the incapacity caused by stroke.

Aqua alba: Also known as lead water, it is water containing lead acetate, similar to aqua vegetomineralis.

Aqua vulneraria: Wound water originally used for washing gunshot wounds that contained comfrey, wormwood, agrimony, and a choice of twenty other ingredients.

Aqua vulneraria viridis: "Wound water" containing aeris viridis (verdigris), the eighteenth-century name for copper acetate, made by placing vinegar in a copper vessel and warming it.

Aqua vulneraria chinata: "Wound water" containing spring water, Peruvian bark, Thedian water, Saturn extract, and ammonium salt.

Armenian bole: The red clay, rich in iron oxide, that is native to Armenia and other regions. It has been used medicinally since ancient times for its drying properties. It was sometimes applied to children's mouths as a remedy for aphthae. The term "bolus" once meant medicinal clay.

Arnica: A flowering plant widespread over most of Europe; it has medicinal properties promoting analgesia and anti-inflammatory effects.

Asafetida: Also spelled asafoetida, it is the dried gum oleoresin found on the taproot of the *Ferula* herb that has had medicinal value since ancient times. Known colloquially as devil's dung.

Ascarides: It is likely that Plenck was referring to pinworms here.

Asturiens: People of Asturias, a region in northwest Spain, who suffered with skin problems that were first described by Gaspar Casal (1681–1759). Casal's description of what was known at the time as Asturian lepra is considered the first description of pellagra.

Atrophic infants: Infants which would today be referred to as having failure to thrive.

Auripigment: Another name for orpiment, the gold-pigmented arsenic sulfide.

Atheromatous: Material similar in appearance to the contents of the atheroma (sebaceous cyst).

Bacchia rosacea: Rosacea of the drunken and jovial, after the Greek god of wine.

Balsam *of Arcaeus*: A liniment named for its inventor, the Spanish physician and surgeon Francesco de Arce (1493–1573), latinized as Arcaeus. It is made from mutton suet (the fat around the kidneys), gum elemi (a tree resin), and common turpentine.

Behen nut oil: The seed oil of *Moringa oleifera*, a tree of the Indian subcontinent and the tropics that is also known as the horseradish tree or drumstick tree. It has been used since ancient times for various medicinal purposes.

Belladonna berries: The berries of *Atropa belladonna*, a poisonous plant that is also known as deadly nightshade and capable of poisoning a person or dog that ingests its berries, leaves, or roots because of the belladonna alkaloids (atropine, hyocyamine, and scopolamine) it contains.

Benzoes: Produced in preparing benzoic acid, by the sublimation of gum benzoin.

Bezoar vinegar: The combination of vinegar and bezoar stones, which were concretions found in the gastrointestinal tracts of animals, long held to have medicinal value.

Bitter salt: Magnesium sulfate, given today externally (Epsom salt, after the British town of Epsom) as a bath salt or internally to manage constipation, certain cardiac arrhythmias, seizures, and pregnancy.

Bittersweet root: *Solanum dulcamara*, the bittersweet nightshade or climbing nightshade.

Black nightshade: *Solanum nigrum.*

Black skin: In the eighteenth century, variance in skin color was considered a consequence of differences in amount of humors in the skin; for example, darker skin contained more black bile than lighter skin.

Blepharitis: Inflammation of skin at base of eyelashes characterized by redness, swelling, itching, scaling, and crusting.

Borsdorf apple: A German dessert apple first cultivated in the twelfth century and used medicinally since the 1500s.

Brambilla: Giovanni Alessandro Brambilla (1728–1800); personal physician of Holy Roman Emperor Joseph II and the first director of the Josephinum in Vienna.

Brazilian pemphigus: Known locally as fogo salvegem, this endemic type of pemphigus (an autoimmune blistering disease) is believed to manifest after the bite of the Simulium black fly which thrives in the vicinity of rural Brazilian rivers.

Buda: Buda and Pest were not unified into Budapest until 1873.

Burdock: Decoctions of the root of this plant have been used in rheumatic, venereal, and other conditions. A traditional herb of the *Arctium* genus, also known as bardan, with many medicinal applications.

Butter from cacao fruit: Cocoa butter; a pale-yellow fat extracted from the cocoa bean.

Cachectic: Having lost significant weight and muscle mass due to disease.

Camphorated: Containing salts formed by the union of the acid of the camphor tree with different bases.

Cancerous: Skin cancer was commonly misdiagnosed as or misnamed herpes in Plenck's era. It is rare for herpes to turn into cancer.

Cancer aquaticus: A severe gangrenous ulceration of the mouth, so-called because of its association with hypersalivation.

Cantharidin/cantharides: Cantharidin, used today as a blistering agent, was taken internally for various medicinal benefits in concentrations as low as 0.005 percent. A medicinal substance utilized since ancient times that is derived from the blister beetle and has aphrodisiacal and blistering properties.

Carbuncle: From the Latin for small coal, it is a cluster of boils.

Carmine: A red dye that comes from the insect known as the cochineal.

Cataplasm: A poultice.

Catarrh: Inflammed mucous membranes of the nasopharynx, leading to runny nose, nasal congestion, and postnasal drip.

Cerate: From Latin *cera*, "wax," it is an externally applied substance that is applied to various skin lesions and has the consistency between an ointment and plaster. It consists of wax, lard, and other medicinal elements.

Ceruse lead: Also known as Venetian ceruse, this skin-whitening agent was made from lead and vinegar and is believed to have the unfortunate consequence of lead poisoning and death.

Chaerophyllum: The rough chervil, used in decoctions along with sarsaparilla for various chronic skin diseases.

Chlorosis: Eighteenth-century term for iron deficiency anemia, which caused a pale green color of the skin.

Coalescence of the eyelids: Inflammation of the sclera, cornea, and conjunctiva was so severe in smallpox that scarring of these parts of the eye were common sequelae among survivors.

Cochlearia: Scurvygrass, an edible herb rich in vitamin C, was used since ancient times as a treatment for scurvy. Formerly *Cochlearia armoracia,* horseradish was also in the past used as a treatment for scurvy.

Cold fever: Plenck is referring to the stage of an illness when the skin is cold and clammy. Cold fever was also a general term for a cold-related malady such as pneumonia and other wintertime ailments. Warm fever referred to maladies associated with heat such as scarlet fever.

Cold water: Before modern times, frostbite was treated with cold water, as opposed to the warm water used today, because of concerns that warm or hot water could precipitate gangrene in affected areas.

Collutorium: A medicated, antiseptic liquid for diseases of the oral cavity.

Comedones: A blackhead or whitehead. A lay term for comedone in this era was worm or grub.

Confirmed syphilis: Or true syphilis, a case of syphilis in the eighteenth or nineteenth centuries (before the advent of serologic testing) that has been confirmed as being syphilis by the physician or surgeon because of classic or pathognomonic physical exam findings.

Contagium: In the eighteenth century and before the germ theory of disease was proven, this ill-defined and general term referred to a substance, such as the "seed of disease" that transferred disease from one person to another. The plague pandemics and other pandemic diseases suggested contagium as a cause of these diseases.

Consumption: Tuberculosis.

Crawly Disease: Translation of "Kriebelkrankheit," the German term for convulsive ergotism, which began with a sensation of running ants upon the limbs and continues with painful contractions of hands and feet. Ergotism is caused by the ingestion of spurred rye, which is rye contaminated with *Claviceps purpurea*, a fungus. Some historical reports associate ergotism with the consumption of radish seeds.

Crinones: Also known as *cridones* and *morgellons*, these lesions were first described in the sixteenth century as a hair-like worm that gives the skin a bristly appearance. The erroneous assumption that these were worms led to two centuries of misunderstanding of their true nature. They are none other than open comedones (blackheads).

Crocus martis: Historically, a naturally occurring red iron oxide or an high iron clay.

Cullen: William Cullen (1710–1790); Edinburgh physician and educator and one of the key figures of the Scottish Enlightenment.

Cuticle: The early modern term for the epidermis. See epidermis.

Cutting the plica: It was widely believed by both the layperson and the medical community of Plenck's era that cutting away the mass of matted hair could be fatal.

Cyprus powder: Fragrant, powdered reindeer moss.

Dancing: In the Italian province of Taranto, a wolf spider bite in the sixteenth and seventeenth centuries triggered a form of hysteria, known as tarantism, in which the victims believed they needed to dance or they would die.

Daniel: Christian Friedrich Daniel (1739–1791); A German nosologist who wrote *Systema aegritudinum* (System of Diseases, 1781) but is most known for editing the final edition of Sauvages' *Nosologia methodica* (1791).

Deadly omen: During the Black Death they were referred to as God's tokens, meaning death was imminent.

Diachylon: A plaster containing lead oxide in a lard and olive oil base.

Diaphoretics: Medications that promote sweating.

Diluents: Medications that increase the proportion of water in the blood.

Dirt: A skin condition that resembles dirt that is difficult to wash off is called terra firma-forme dermatosis.

Dogfish: A type of small shark that is considered a delicacy in Germany and consumed in other parts of Europe. The dogfish contains too much methylmercury to be consumed on a regular basis (more than twice per month).

Dracunculus: Under modern taxonomy, *Dracunculus medinensis*, or the Guinea worm, is the longest nematode that affects humans. Known to exist since ancient times, the worm enters the body in its larval stage as the host ingests contaminated water. The adult form then migrates from the wall of the intestinal tract to the skin, causing a blister on the skin, which contains the emerging head of the rather long worm (70–120 cm). Traditionally, it was extracted from the body by piercing the emerging head with a wooden stick, and then twisting the worm on the stick a little each day, being careful not to pull too hard and risk breaking it off in the body. The World Health Organization hopes to eradicate it by 2030.

Dram: 1/8 of an ounce; a unit of weight for apothecaries.

Dropsy: Edema, or the accumulation of fluid in the tissues, classically associated with heart failure.

Ear finger: The little finger, with which we usually pick the ear.

Earwax: Earwax was used since ancient times for various dermatological purposes including bites and wounds.

Elephantiasis: Until the modern era, this ancient term referred to the condition we now call Hansen's disease. From Plenck's description, his elephantiasis is more in line with the modern use of the word. Elephantiasis in the modern sense refers to a condition in which the lower legs and feet enlarge in size and the skin thickens, due to a variety of lymphatic disorders.

Elixir: A sweet, flavored liquid, usually containing alcohol, used to mask the taste of medication.

English plaster: A paste of ground mustard and flour mixed with warm water, then applied to fabric and placed on the body for medicinal effects; it included animal products like blood or urine as well as beer or whiskey.

Enula: A tall Eurasian herb whose roots are used medicinally.

Epidermis: The top (outermost layer) of skin.

Epinyctis: From the Greek for "upon the night," a pustule that rises in the night and forms a painful inflammatory tumor of a livid color. Perhaps a bug bite or skin infection is the cause.

Erythema: Redness of the skin brought about by inflammation, as opposed to flushing or some other cause of redness.

Erythema ab igne: A term still used today that refers to the net-like pattern of hyperpigmentation and erythema caused by chronic external heat sources directed toward the skin, such as space heaters, heating pads, and laptops.

Eschar: A dry, dark scab.

Esserae: Obsolete term, possibly representing a larger, flatter form of hives or urticarial dermatitis.

Ethiopian minerals: A black mercury sulfide.

Exophytic flesh: Exuberant granulation tissue (also known as a pyogenic granuloma) which not uncommonly arises as a complication of ingrown nails. The word "exophytic" means growing outward.

Exostosis: Bony outgrowth emerging from a bone.

Exutorio: An ulcer that is artificially induced and maintained for healing purposes.

Face spared: It is true that scabies in the modern sense does not involve the face.

Fasting saliva: The saliva in one's mouth upon first awakening was considered to have therapeutic value for centuries.

Farina: Flour or meal-like matter.

Favus: From the Latin word for honeycomb, favus refers to a type of tinea (tinea favosa), caused by *Trichophyton schoenleinii,* which is characterized by cup-shaped crusts that cluster together to form a honeycomb appearance.

Feign disease: As in Munchausen syndrome.

Flammula jovis: A plant, also known as Upright Virgin's Bower (*Clematis recta*) whose flowers and leaves when applied to the skin produce inflammation and vesication, desired effects in treating condyloma.

Flesh fly: Egg-laying flies that deposit eggs on carrion, dung, decaying material, or open wounds of mammals.

Flowers of zinc: Also known as philosopher's wool, it refers to zinc oxide obtained as a light white insoluble powder by burning zinc. Used as an antiseptic and astringent preparation and for making zinc ointment.

Fonticulus: An artificial sore made by a puncture and kept open with a pea for the purpose of obtaining a discharge.

Freckle of pregnancy: Melasma in the modern sense, the mask-like hyperpigmentation of the face that affects pregnant women.

Fumariae: An herb that has been used medicinally since the Middle Ages, including for dermatologic conditions; contains fumaric acid, used in present day in both psoriasis and multiple sclerosis. The juice of this plant is used in diseases of the skin, such as leprosy.

Fumigation: The process of generating fumes of boiling herbs and other ingredients, usually emanating from a bowl under the seated patient, for therapeutic purposes. The fumes are breathed in or penetrate into the skin.

Furia infernali: *Furia infernali* was first described by the Swedish physician and naturalist Carl Linnaeus but was later determined to be a figment of his imagination.

Good-king-henry: A medicinal spinach-like plant, sometimes called wild spinach, grown for its juicy and flavorful arrow-shaped leaves.

Haemeropathos: Morning or daytime suffering.

Hartmann: Francis Xavier Hartmann (unknown dates)**:** Viennese botanist who recorded a botanical classification system.

Hectic fever: A recurring fever with chills and sweats associated with a chronic wasting disease such as tuberculosis. It later came to mean any intermittent fever that has wide swings in temperature.

Hellebore: A poisonous plant that has been used medicinally since ancient times. It was the first source of resveratrol which was discovered in 1939.

Hirudo: Leeches.

Hydatid: A fluid-filled cyst.

Hydrops: Severe swelling of a particular area.

Ichor: A watery discharge from a sore or blister.

Ignis sacer: "Holy fire," an ancient term that referred to several different painful skin diseases over the centuries, including erysipelas, ergotism, and zoster.

Impetigo benigna: Plenck appears to be describing psoriasis. Impetigo did not come to mean what it means today until the nineteenth century. Impetigo was a term for psoriasis dating back to the time of Celsus (first century CE).

Impetigo retropulsa: Morbid matter from impetigo going into the body and causing internal disease.

Infarction: Obstruction of blood flow to a part of the body.

Infused nicotianae: The tobacco plant, *Nicotiana tabacum*, indigenous to the Americas, was first brought to Europe in the sixteenth century. Named after Jean Nicot de Villemain (1530–1604), who first brought tobacco leaves and seeds to Paris. Infused means the tobacco was soaked in a liquid such as water.

Iliac crests: The protruding portions of the hip bones bilaterally located on the lower back.

India: Eighteenth-century term for the part of the world beyond the Indus river.

Inoculation: Also known as variolation, this method involved introducing smallpox pustular matter into the skin of non-immune persons in order to induce immunity. Variolation was the primary means of preventing smallpox in the era before Jenner's introduction of vaccination (1796) and had the risk of inflicting full-blown smallpox in 1 out of 50.

Internal lice: The ancients, medievals, and early moderns all believed that lice were generated from morbid humors from within the body and expelled onto the skin. This theory of spontaneous generation was disproven by Francisco Redi (1626–1697), but it took over a century for the debunking to be fully adopted.

Intertrigo: A modern term, which means skin rash of a fold of the body, such as underarm, inframammary area, or groin, and it's caused by friction, heat, and moisture.

Iron: It is extraordinary that replacing iron was known in Plenck's time to be an effective treatment for nail problems related to anemia. We know today that the main nail manifestation of iron deficiency anemia is "spoon nails" (koilonycia).

Jugular glands: Cervical lymph nodes.

Lanugo: Fine hair that covers a fetus or newborn.

Lapathum acutum: A historical name for the dock, a plant used medicinally for centuries.

Lapis causticus: Fused sodium or potassium hydroxide. *Lapis* is Latin for stone but also an alchemical term for non-volatile solids.

Lapis infernalis: Also known as "lunar caustic," the "infernal stone" refers to silver nitrate used as a cautery.

Larvae aestrorum: It is the authors' view that Plenck meant "larva oestrorum." *Oestres* was a genus of botflies known at the time to infest cattle. There is no reference to "aestrorum" in any other text contemporary with Plenck's. Or he might have meant "summer larva" from the Latin for summer, aestas.

Lepra: During Plenck's time, the word "lepra" referred to a variety of chronic skin diseases that included Hansen's disease and psoriasis.

Leuce: Obsolete term for a skin disease of questionable identity but that was characterized by white spots on the skin; possibly vitiligo.

Lice: Physicians in the eighteenth century and prior believed in spontaneous generation, the idea that lice and other organisms could arise on the body not as offspring of similar organisms, but spontaneously. Lice are not known to cluster under the skin inside blisters.

Limoniums: Also known as sea lavender or marsh-rosemary, these are flowering plants of the *Plumbaginaceae* family (leadwort or plumbago family).

Linaria: Plant whose seeds were frequently used as a cataplasm or poultice.

Lines: Two lines is equal to 1/6 of an inch (1 line is 1/12 of an inch).

Linnaeus: Carl Linnaeus (1707–1778); Swedish physician, botanist, and zoologist who classified living things using a binomial nomenclature in *Systema naturae* (1735).

Liver spot: Referred to as liver spot because they have the same color as liver and the cause of these spots was believed to be excessive bile.

Liver of antimony: A preparation of antimony that has the color of liver and that is created from the explosive reaction of putting fire to a compound of antimony and saltpeter.

Liver of Sulfur: A mixture of potassium sulfide, potassium polysulfide, potassium thiosulfate, and potassium bisulfide that was taken orally for various medicinal purposes.

Livor: Blue or purplish discoloration of the skin.

Locust-eaters: A tribe in Ethiopia called the Acridophagi (locust-eaters) were believed since the time of Pliny (first century CE) to subsist on locusts.

Lorry: Anne-Charles Lorry (1726–1783); French physician who is widely considered the first French dermatologist and the author of *Tractatus de Morbis Cutaneis* (1777).

Lovage*:* *Levisticum officinale*, a perennial herbaceous plant.

Lumbricus effractore: The navel worm, or umbilical worm, was an intestinal worm that was believed to emerge from the navel. "Effractore" is from the Latin for burglar.

Lunula: The half-moon shaped white spot at the proximal end of normal nails.

Lupin seeds: The yellow-brown legume seeds of the genus *Lupinus*.

Lycopodia: *Lycopodium clavatum*, a clubmoss, used medicinally since ancient times and up until present day. It can be consumed as a tea or drops internally, or applied externally as a compress.

Macbride: David Macbride (1726–1778); Irish physician and nosologist who wrote *A Methodological Introduction to the Theory and Practice of Physic* (1772).

Macula lata Plateri: Wide spots of Platter," first described by Felix Platter (1536–1614) in *Praxis Medica*. Plenck's description states this is another term for ignis sacer (erysipelas). The original description of Platter discusses blue lesions in the setting of fever: "I saw a girl stricken with the disease eight days before, delirious, with such a clamor that it filled and stirred the whole neighborhood. Her parents said she complained only of heartache, her pulse weak and not very rapid. And what is worthy of note, a black-blue spot appeared under the right nipple on her chest, so wide that it was not raised, I predicted her death, which also followed the next day. I suspected it was a pestilential or malignant fever, which was then raging in the neighborhood. In 1596, when it had left us the previous year, it was still manifesting itself in her." Later authors questioned whether Platter was discussing anthrax.

Magisterio of bismuth: Bismuth subnitrate, or white bismuth.

Malignant fever: Yellow fever.

Malignant ulcer: Melanoma that looks like a lentigo at first and then evolves rather slowly into a more obvious melanoma, which eventually ulcerates.

Malis: Obsolete term for a skin lesion believed to contain insects or worms.

Malpighian mucus: Obsolete term for the deep germinative layer of the epidermis, including the stratum basale and stratum spinosum.

Mamapian: Or *mama pian*, mother yaws (the largest lesion of yaws). Yaws is one of the three non-venereal treponematoses, which are tropical diseases closely related to syphilis.

Mars balls: Prepared by boiling iron filings and potassium hydrogen tartrate in water, the product of which was formed into balls and placed in bath water.

Martial: Referring to iron (the god of war, Mars, was associated with iron); sourish iron water with tartarized iron and aromatics (see mars balls); a type of mineral water with a high concentration of iron oxide.

Masterwort: *Imperatoria ostruthium*; a flowering plant with roots and leaves that have been used in traditional Austrian medicine internally and externally.

Mastiche: A resin produced by the mastic tree (*Pistacia lentiscus*), first discussed medicinally in the Hippocratic corpus.

Melas: An obsolete term for a form of leprosy that caused depressed dark spots in the skin. Leprosy had disappeared from Europe by 1600 but was known by Europeans to be endemic in Arabia and given the name "leprosy of the Arabs."

Melasma: Plenck's description is suggestive of a modern diagnosis of chronic venous stasis, with its tendency to darken the skin and eventuate into leg ulcers. It could also refer to melanoma. The modern use of the word "melasma" refers to the pigmentary condition that involves the face.

Mercurial milk: A preparation of mercury that was as white as milk. Could also refer to the crushed plant material of the *Mercurialis* herb blended with water and whey, resulting in spontaneous lactic acid.

Mercurius gummosus: A form of mercury invented by Plenck that mixed mercury with acacia gum that could treat syphilis without the salivation induced by the mercury.

Mercurius vivus: Quicksilver, elemental mercury.

Mercury sublimate: Applied in the form of a lotion to venereal sores and given internally in small quantities in the eighteenth century management of syphilis.

Mesenteric: In this case, intestinal, but the word can refer to the mesentery, a portion of the peritoneum which attaches the stomach, small intestine, pancreas, spleen, and other organs to the posterior wall of the abdomen.

Metal dross: The waste product removed from molten metal during the smelting process.

Miasma: Refers to the "bad air" believed to cause infectious diseases before germ theory was proven in the nineteenth century.

Miliary fever: Miliary fever referred nonspecifically to any febrile illness that was associated with miliaria, which are red papules that erupt because of blocked sweat ducts in the setting of the sweats of fever. It was the cause of death of Plenck's neighbor, Wolfgang Amadeus Mozart.

Mulatto: An outdated term for a person of mixed African and European ancestry.

Morpiones: An obsolete term for lice.

Mykonos: A Greek island in the Aegean Sea known for its bald men since the time of Strabo (64 BCE–24 CE), the ancient Greek geographer who first wrote about them.

Myrmecial: A type of palmoplantar wart.

Nasturtium: A flowering plant (*Tropaeolum*) that produces an oil. A remedy containing nasturtium and horseradish root is an effective antibiotic for sinusitis and urinary tract infections in the modern era.

Neapolitan ointment*:* A mercury-containing ointment.

Needle causes no pain: Lesions of Hansen's disease are characteristically anesthetic because the infection damages the Schwann cells of peripheral nerves. Anesthesia was known to be a feature of Hansen's disease since the Middle Ages.

Nigritae: People living along the Niger river.

Noli me tangere: "Touch me not" was the primary term for skin cancer in the modern sense for hundreds of years. It was widely believed that surgical intervention of these types of skin lesions only made matters worse for the patient, presumably because the concept of clear margins of surgical excision of cancer had not yet been realized.

Noma: A term still used today for an oral ulcerative disease associated with malnutrition which has a description not very different from Plenck's.

Nymphs: Eighteenth-century term for labia minora.

Oil of scorpion: Made by cooking scorpions in oil and straining the liquid from the solid, to which various ingredients were added.

Oil of spike: A type of lavender oil made from the whole plant and not just the blossoms.

Ointment of frogs: An ointment made from the fat of green frogs.

Oil of tartar per deliquium: Another term for potassium carbonate, a salt produced by the calcination of tartar (potassium bitartrate) that liquifies in the humidity of the open atmosphere.

Orpiment: Arsenic sulfide.

Ophthalmia: ighteenth-century term for conjunctivitis.

Otorrhea: Ear drainage.

Ox gall: Ox bile, the fluid obtained from the gallbladder of the ox, used medicinally since the days of ancient Chinese medicine and still consumed as a supplement in pill form today.

Oxycrate: A mixture of water and vinegar softened with honey.

Oxymel: A mixture of vinegar and honey.

Panaritii bullosa: Whitlow or felon; paronychia.

Pannonian: Region now occupied by Hungary, East Austria, and former Yugoslavia.

Paresis: Partial paralysis.

Patagones: The peoples living in the southern part of South America, rumored by explorers such as Magellan to be giants with "big feet," but they left big footprints because of the mocassins they wore.

Periscelis: A leg band worn by women around thigh or ankle, that is, a garter.

Peruvian bark: A historically important natural remedy discovered by Jesuits missionaries in Peru in the 1620s. Referring to the bark of the cinchona tree, Peruvian bark was used as a cure-all for fevers. It was later determined to contain quinine, a treatment for malaria.

Petechiae: Punctate hemorrhages in the skin with a wide variety of causes, such as low platelets.

Pernio: Both pernio and chilblains are still terms used today, and refer to tender, purpuric macules and papules brought about by exposure of the digits to the cold.

Pica: The desire to eat something not typically eaten, such as clay, plaster, or ice.

Phagedenic water: A caustic made from quick lime (calcium oxide) and corrosive sublimate (mercury bichloride) used primarily to remove proud flesh (granulation tissue) and gangrenous tissue.

Phalange: bone of the finger.

Phimosis: Phimosis is a state of the penis in which the foreskin cannot be retracted, while a paraphimosis occurs when the foreskin is stuck in a retracted position.

Phthisis: Eighteenth-century term for tuberculosis.

Pitch depilatory: A potentially ghastly eighteenth- and nineteenth-century approach to treating tinea in which pitch was applied to the scalp and then removed vigorously from the scalp for the purposes of epilating infected hairs. A risk of the procedure was partial or complete avulsion (traumatic removal) of the scalp.

Pitch oil: Pine resin or extraction of fir trees.

Platula: An obsolete term for lice.

Plethoric: Full of blood.

Plica polonica: Also known as trichoma, plica polonica was a cultural phenomenon that started in Poland in the seventeenth century but occurred in other parts of Europe. These patients developed a mass of irreversibly matted hair, believed to be associated with a variety of internal manifestations, and according to both physicians of the era and the afflicted, removal could lead to death.

Pliny: As described by Pliny the Elder in his *Historia naturalis* (77 CE), mentagra was a skin disease that preferentially erupted on the face of Roman aristocratic men who were utterly devastated by the disfigurement. Pliny's mentagra was very likely equivalent to a staphylococcal skin infection of the face (impetigo or folliculitis barbae).

Plumaciol: A soft pad of wool or cotton used on wounds.

Porrum: A wart that resembles the flowers of the leek (*Allium porrum*).

Primis viis: The first way or passage, that is, the gastrointestinal tract.

Proximate cause: The immediate cause of a disease. The underlying cause is often referred to as the remote cause or exciting cause of a disease.

Ptyalism: Hypersalivation, the excessive output of saliva that accompanies mercury toxicity.

Pubic lice: Pubic lice are known to infest the eyelashes.

Publicus ordinarius: The highest rank of a professor; equivalent to full professor or professor with chair.

Purulent: Containing or exuding pus.

Putrid fever: A fever deemed to be caused by putrefaction of the blood and considered more serious than other fevers; by the late eighteenth century, putrid fever became synonymous with typhus.

Red precipitate: Mercuric oxide (HgO).

Retrograde scabies: It was believed that disease of the skin could be driven inward if not handled properly, and this was undesirable. Scabies going inward.

Rhus tree: *Toxicodendron vernicifluum*, also known by the common name Chinese lacquer tree or *Rhus vernificera*, is a tree found in China, Japan, and Korea that contains an urushiol resin (the same as in poison ivy and sumac) which when dried serves as a lacquer for lacquerware such as dishes, furniture, and coffins.

Ricinus: The castor oil plant.

Sabadilla: A plant of the lilly family and a homeopathic remedy for worms.

Sac. Caes. Reg. Apost. Maj.: Brambilla's military rank abbreviated. Translated as Sacred, Imperial, Royal, Apostolic, and Majestic.

Sagar: Johann Baptiste Michael Sagar (1702–1778); Viennese physician who classified diseases in his "System of symptomatic diseases" (1771).

Sarcomas: Eighteenth-century term for a fleshy tumor on any part of the body. Today, it refers to a malignant tumor of the muscle, bone, or connective tissue.

Salt of tartar: Potassium carbonate.

Saponaria: A family of flowering plants commonly known as soapworts.

Sarmatia: A historical eastern European and western Asian region that now contains parts of Russia, Ukraine, and the neighboring Asian nations.

Sarsaparilla: A tropical, climbing woody vine used since ancient times to treat conditions like arthritis, syphilis, and various skin conditions.

Saturnine: Containing lead acetate. Lead acetate water, similar to aqua vegetamineralis. Salt of Saturn is synonymous with lead acetate.

Sauvages: François Boissier de Sauvages de Lacroix (1706–1767), A trailblazing French physician and botanist who organized the first general classification of diseases (nosology) in 1731.

Savin powder: A powder from the shrub *Juniper sabina* that has caustic properties when applied to the skin.

Scarification: Incising the skin with a lancet in order to cause scar tissue.

Scolopendra forficulata: A centipede which can get into the ear.

Scrofula: Occurs in the neck when tuberculous infection spreads out of the upper lobe of the lung and into the lymph nodes of the supraclavicular region, which subsequently suppurate, erode, and drain onto the surface of the skin.

Scurvy: Known today to be caused by vitamin C deficiency, scurvy killed millions in the sixteenth through eighteenth centuries and was characterized by weakness, fatigue, sore arms and legs, anemia, gum disease, easy bruising, poor wound healing, personality changes, and death from infection or bleeding.

Sebaceous tumor: The epidermal inclusion cyst (sebaceous cyst) in the modern sense.

Sebum: The oil released onto the surface of the skin from the sebaceous glands; the material trapped in the pores of teenagers with acne.

Sex organs: In reference to the extremely high libido, termed Satyrism, that was classically associated with lepra.

Sirones: The early modern term for the tiny mite that was found on the digits of persons afflicted with *the itch*, now known to be the scabies mite. Though discovered and postulated to be the actual cause of *the itch* by Bonomo in the seventeenth century, it was not until the mid-nineteenth century that the scabies mite was widely accepted as the cause of scabies. The word is derived from the French word, *ciron*, for the itch mite.

Silesia: A historical central European region that is now a part of Poland, Czechia, and Germany.

Solution of sublimated mercury: Another name for corrosive sublimate (mercuric chloride).

Spermatic function: Unclear meaning of the word *spermaticis* and the phrase is missing from the German translation, but inferring from the final sentence of the section, it is possible that Plenck was referring to males who masturbate, or perhaps the opposite, that is, those who produce sperm but do not release it. Both masturbation and seminal continence have been linked to acne since the time of Plenck.

Sphacelus: An obsolete term for gangrene.

Spina ventosa: Tuberculosis of the phalanges, also known as tuberculous dactylitis.

Spines of the tibia: Bony ridge on anterior surface of the tibia.

Spirit of ligni sancti: Guaiacum, a flowering tree native to the Americas that was imported in Europe in the sixteenth century and contained a resin that was purported to treat syphilis.

Spirit of nitre: Another name for aqua forti (solution of nitric acid in water).

Spirit of salt: Hydrochloric acid.

Spirit of wine: Ethanol.

Staphisagria: Commonly known as stavesacre, it was a plant used as a pediculocide as far back as ancient Greece, and it contains an alkaloid that is indeed insecticidal.

Stensen's salivary ducts: The opening of the parotid duct, which lies on the inside of the buccal cheek across from the second upper molar tooth.

Strengthening agents: A wide variety of medicinal herbs that were believed to strengthen various organs.

Sudamina: Retained today as a modern word for miliaria crystallina.

Sweet mercury: Mercury chloride, calomel.

Sweet spirit of salt: Spirit of wine and spirit of salt (hydrochloric acid) mixed together and distilled.

Sympathetic remedies: Treatments intended to heal a wound, injury or skin problem from afar, without ever touching the wound or skin. Examples include the weapon salve, which healed a wound when it was applied to the weapon rather than a wound, and vitriol powder, which healed a wound when the dressing from the wound was applied to the powder.

Syrup of spina cervina: *Rhamnus cathartica*, the berries of which (buckthorn berries) were once used as a cathartic (purgative).

Tamarind whey: The edible fruit of the leguminous tamarind tree was boiled in milk and used as a laxative.

Tartars: A Turkic-speaking people from the steppes of Russia who joined the forces of the Mongol conqueror Genghis Khan (thirteenth century), eventually leading to the term "Tartar" (or Tatar) becoming synonymous with Mongols.

Terminth: A swelling or tumor with a black pustule resembling the fruit of the turpentine tree.

Terminthi neonatorum: Neonatal pemphigus according to Ferdinand von Hebra. Other possibilities are childhood bullous dermatosis and bullous impetigo.

Thapsia: *Thapsia garganica*, the deadly carrot, which has a long history of medicinal application and contains a substance called thapsigargin, which may have antiviral and anti-cancer properties.

Thedian water: A type of *aqua vulneraria*, "wound water" that is applied to wounds and that contains vinegar water, spirit of wine (wine distilled down to purified ethanol), spirits of vitriol (dilute sulfuric acid), and white sugar.

Invented by Johann Christian Theden (1714–1797), a Prussian surgeon and personal physician of Frederick the Great (1712–1786).

Theriac: A medical concoction and panacea containing a variety of therapeutic ingredients, including roots, stems, barks, leaves, flowers, seeds, gums, oils, resins, animal parts, and minerals.

Tinea: The modern word "tinea" comes from the Latin, *tinea*, which means a gnawing worm that eats holes in an everyday object.

Tinea unguium: A term used today to denote "corruption" of the nail plate specifically by a fungus; the cause of this condition was not known in Plenck's time.

Tophi: Plural of tophus, a deposit of uric acid crystals in the skin of patients with gout.

True skin: The dermis. Physicians have long believed the dermis to be the true skin, and the epidermis (or cuticle) to be simply a layer generated by the true skin. The sixteenth-century surgeon Ambroise Pare even referred to the epidermis as the "bastard skin."

Tsömör: Or csömör, it refers to an exhausting febrile illness endemic in Hungary in the eighteenth century.

Tuberculosis: Known as the white death or white plague, tuberculosis and its associated anemia of chronic disease caused a general pallor of the skin.

Turpentine oil: A fluid obtained by distilling the resin of several pine trees.

Two-headed snake: A reference to *amphibaenas*, a footless, worm-like lizard of Brazil with a head at one end and a tail that looked like another head at the other end. The locals attributed their pemphigus (fogo salvagem) to these "two-headed snakes" but it may actually result from the bite of the black fly, given the higher incidence of this type of pemphigus near rivers and streams that the black fly inhabits.

Tyrian: From Tyrus, a serpent oft-mentioned in medieval encyclopedias. The word "theriac" might be derived from it, as the venom of tyrus, which was very poisonous, was often used in small amounts as an antidote to poisons.

Tyriasis: One of several historical terms for what is now called Hansen's disease.

Unguent: A general term for a semisolid substance applied externally to the skin. An ointment is a greasy type of unguent.

Uritides: The nocturnal form is not different from epinyctis. From the description, Plenck was likely describing bug bites (given lack of pus) or a nodular form of scabies, or less likely, some type of skin infection (which would contain pus). See epinyctis.

Variegated skin: While one could speculate that Plenck's observed oddity might result from severe bruising, there is no known skin disease that can produce these color changes.

Vegetomineral water: Water fortified with lead acetate.

Venetian soap: Soap compounded from sodium hydroxide and olive oil. It can be molded into hard soap but dissolved in water. Now known as white castile soap.

Vesicatory: A chemical agent that when applied on the skin causes a blister.

Vibices: Plural of vibex, it refers to the presence of linear purpura; a seldom used term.

Vinegar of squill: Solution of sea onion (or sea squill, a land plant) and vinegar used medicinally for centuries.

Viper broth: Broth prepared from dried flesh of viper that was used since the time of Galen.

Virginia snakeroot: A New World plant used for medicinal purposes in Europe in the eighteenth century, especially for ague (malaria).

Virus: Viruses were not discovered until the twentieth century, but the term was used synonymously with contagion in early modern medicine.

Vitriol: Sulfuric acid.

Vogel: Rudolf Augustin Vogel (1724–1774); German professor of medicine at the University of Gottingen, who published a nosology entitled *Definitiones generum morborum*, (Definitions of the Kinds of Diseases, 1764).

War: The Seven Years' War (1756–1763), the main belligerents of which were Austria and Britain versus Prussia and France.

Water drinkers: A reminder of the old adage, "moderation in all things." In Plenck's view, too much water or too much wine could both lead to rosacea.

White precipitated mercury: Also known as calomel.

Wild pansy: *Viola tricolor*, a European wild flower used in herbal medicine for skin diseases and eczema.

Wild radish: It was believed that consuming wild radish seeds (*Raphanus raphanistrum*) could cause a convulsive disease, resembling ergotism. The Germans called it "Krabelkrankheiten." See Crawly disease.

Winteran bark: The red-brown bark of a tree (*Drimys winteri*) that was used primarily as a preventative and treatment for scurvy in the Age of Exploration. It was first discovered in South America by one of Sir Francis Drake's men, John Wynter (1555–1638).

White vitriol: Another name for zinc sulfate; white vitriol is one of several types of vitriol, which are inorganic substances containing a sulfate group.

Whitlow: An infection of the distal finger, often purulent or blistery.

ABOUT THE AUTHORS

Scott M. Jackson, MD, earned his medical degree from Louisiana State University Health Sciences Center in New Orleans. He is a physician-historian, adjunct faculty at the Alice L. Walton School of Medicine, and a dermatologist in private practice in Northwest Arkansas. He has authored a complete history of dermatology entitled *Skin Disease and the History of Dermatology: Order Out of Chaos* (2023). He lives in Bentonville, Arkansas.

Althea C. Ashe, PhD, earned her master's degree in Greek and Latin from Louisiana State University and a doctorate in Latin Education from the University of Georgia. In addition to teaching Latin for 31 years, she was the director of Specialized Language Instruction in Latin from 2001 until her retirement in 2011. She resides in Baton Rouge, Louisiana.

ACKNOWLEDGMENTS

The authors would like to thank Richard LaFleur, Johanna Sandrock, Deborah MacInnes, and Kurt Krottendorfer for sharing their expertise, suggestions, advice, and support along the way.

www.ingramcontent.com/pod-product-compliance
Ingram Content Group UK Ltd.
Pitfield, Milton Keynes, MK11 3LW, UK
UKHW042236260226
468429UK00003B/15

9 781839 999369